THE ADRENAL INSUFFICIENCY HANDBOOK

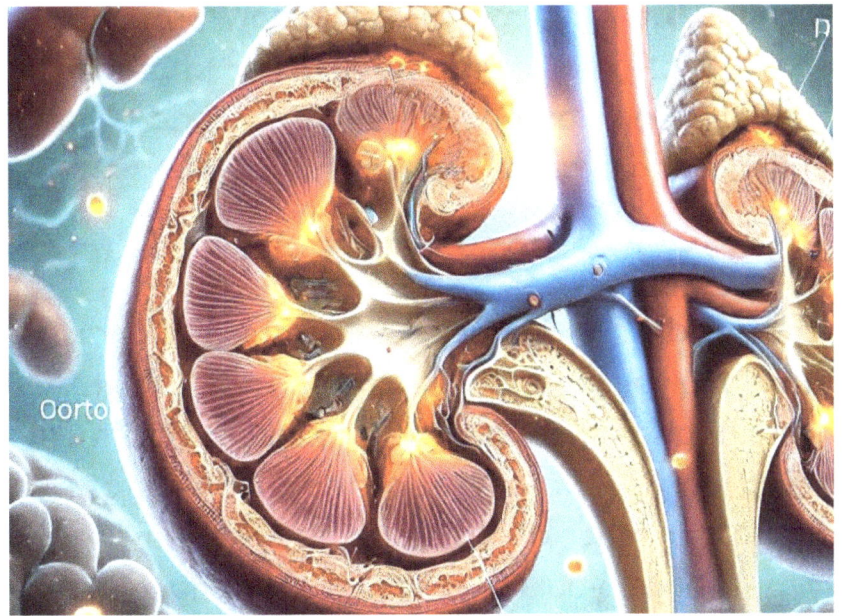

Understanding, Managing and Thriving with Addison's Disease, Low Cortisol and Adrenal Fatigue

Written by Jeffrey C Lawson

Copyright © 2024 All Rights Reserved

No part of this book may be reproduced, stored in a retrieval system, or transmitted in any form or by any means—electronic, mechanical, photocopying, recording, or otherwise—without prior written permission from the publisher/author.

Disclaimer:

This book is intended for informational and educational purposes only. It is not a substitute for professional medical advice, diagnosis, treatment or medications. Always seek the advice of your physician or other qualified healthcare provider with any questions you may have regarding a medical condition. The author and publisher disclaim any liability for actions taken based on the content of this book.

Table of Content

Part 1: Introduction and Overview   **6**
  Definition and Explanation   6
  History of Adrenal Insufficiency   7
  Importance of Adrenal Glands   10
  Book Objectives and Scope   13
  Target Audience   15

Part 2: Anatomy and Physiology   **18**
  Adrenal Gland Anatomy   18
  Hormones Produced by Adrenal Glands   20
  Regulation of Adrenal Function   22
  Adrenal Gland Disorders   25
  Physiological Effects of Adrenal Hormones   27

Part 3: Types of Adrenal Insufficiency   **30**
  Primary Adrenal Insufficiency (Addison's Disease)   30
  Secondary Adrenal Insufficiency   33
  Tertiary Adrenal Insufficiency   37
  Congenital Adrenal Hyperplasia (CAH)   40
  Adrenal Crisis   44

Part 4: Causes and Risk Factors   **50**
  Genetic Causes   50
  Autoimmune Disorders   52
  Infections   55
  Trauma and Surgery   57

Medication and Substances	59
Other Medical Conditions	62
Part 5: Symptoms and Diagnosis	**66**
Clinical Presentation	66
Physical Examination	69
Laboratory Tests	71
Differential Diagnosis	75
Part 6: Treatment and Management	**78**
Glucocorticoid Replacement Therapy	78
Mineralocorticoid Replacement Therapy	81
Adrenal Androgen Replacement Therapy	85
Surgery and Radiation Therapy	88
Lifestyle Modifications	92
Emergency Management	95
Part 7: Special Considerations	**100**
Pediatric Adrenal Insufficiency	100
Adrenal Insufficiency in Pregnancy	104
Adrenal Insufficiency in Elderly	108
Psychological and Emotional Aspects	112
Traveling and Vaccination Considerations	116
Part 8: Complications and Prognosis	**120**
Short Term Complications	120
Long Term Complications	123
Prognosis and Quality of Life	126
Future Directions	129
Part 9: Appendices	**132**

Glossary of Terms	132
Resources and Support Groups	137
Medication Lists	141
Laboratory Test Reference Ranges	145
Emergency Protocol	149

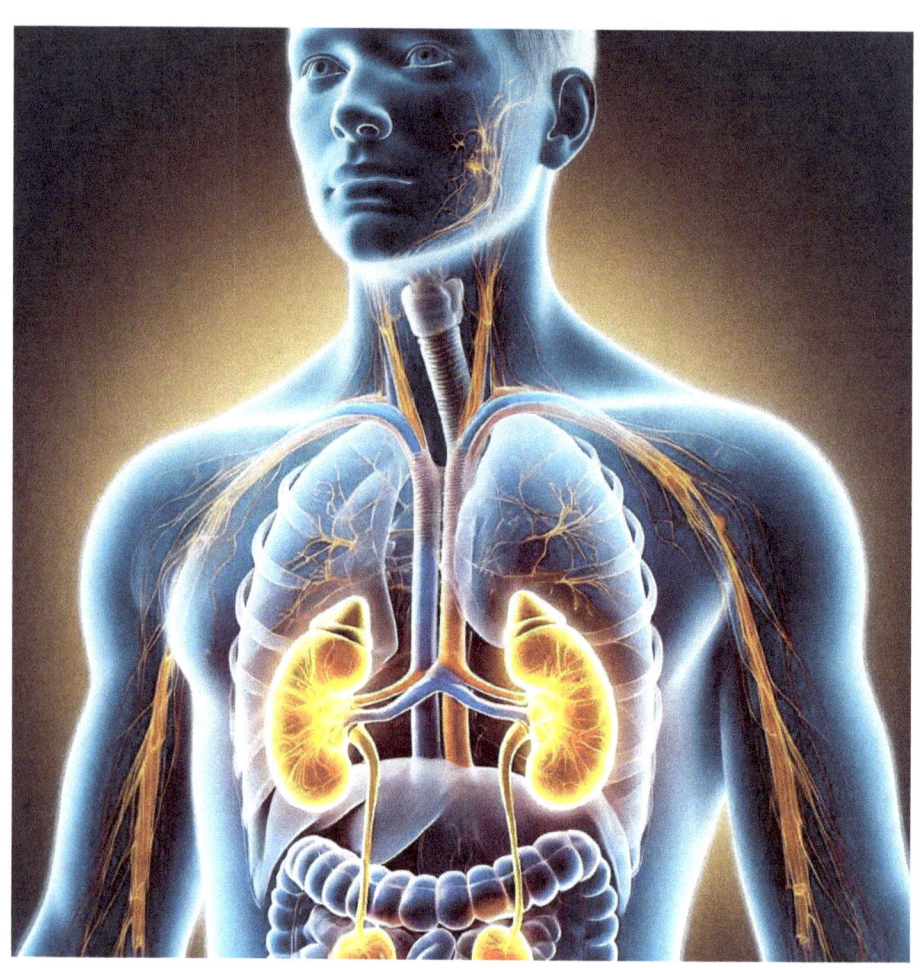

Part 1: Introduction and Overview

Definition and Explanation

Adrenal insufficiency is a rare disorder that occurs when your adrenal glands don't produce enough of the hormone cortisol. The adrenal glands are small, triangular-shaped glands that sit on top of your kidneys. They produce several hormones, including cortisol, which helps your body respond to stress, regulate blood sugar levels, and maintain blood pressure.

There are two main types of adrenal insufficiency:

- Primary adrenal insufficiency: Also known as Addison's disease, this occurs when the adrenal glands themselves are damaged and can't produce enough cortisol.
- Secondary adrenal insufficiency: This occurs when the pituitary gland, which is located at the base of your brain, doesn't produce enough of the hormone ACTH (adrenocorticotropic hormone). ACTH

stimulates the adrenal glands to produce cortisol.

Symptoms of adrenal insufficiency can vary depending on the severity of the condition. Common symptoms include fatigue, muscle weakness, weight loss, and low blood pressure. In severe cases, adrenal insufficiency can lead to an adrenal crisis, which is a life-threatening condition that requires immediate medical attention.

Adrenal insufficiency is usually treated with hormone replacement therapy, which involves taking medication to replace the cortisol that your body is not producing. The type and dosage of medication will depend on your individual needs.

History of Adrenal Insufficiency

The history of adrenal insufficiency is long and fascinating, with roots dating back to ancient times. While the specific condition wasn't fully understood until the 20th century, early physicians recognized the symptoms and effects of adrenal gland dysfunction.

Ancient Times and Early Observations

In ancient Egypt, the Ebers Papyrus (circa 1550 BC) describes a condition characterized by weakness, weight loss, and darkening of the skin, which are now recognized as classic symptoms of adrenal insufficiency. However, at the time, these symptoms were often attributed to various other causes.

19th Century: A Turning Point

The 19th century marked a significant turning point in the understanding of adrenal insufficiency. In 1855, Thomas Addison, a British physician, described a case series of patients with a syndrome characterized by weakness, fatigue, weight loss, and a bronze-like skin pigmentation. This syndrome, now known as Addison's disease, is a form of primary adrenal insufficiency.

20th Century: Unraveling the Mystery

The 20th century brought about significant advancements in the understanding of adrenal insufficiency. Researchers began to unravel the complex hormonal interactions involved in adrenal function. In the early 1900s, scientists discovered that the adrenal glands produce a variety of hormones, including cortisol, which plays a crucial role in regulating stress response, metabolism, and immune function.

The development of hormone replacement therapy in the mid-20th century revolutionized the treatment of adrenal insufficiency. Corticosteroid medications, such as hydrocortisone and prednisone, became available to replace the missing cortisol and improve the quality of life for patients with this condition.

Modern Era: Ongoing Research and Advances

In recent decades, research has continued to expand our understanding of adrenal insufficiency. Scientists have identified genetic mutations that can cause primary adrenal insufficiency and have developed more precise diagnostic tests. Additionally, advancements in medical technology have led to improved treatment options and better monitoring of patients with adrenal insufficiency.

While significant progress has been made, challenges remain. Adrenal insufficiency is a complex condition that can be difficult to diagnose, especially in its early stages. Moreover, long-term treatment with hormone replacement therapy requires careful monitoring to prevent side effects and ensure optimal health.

Despite these challenges, the future of adrenal insufficiency research is promising. Ongoing research aims to develop more targeted therapies, improve diagnostic accuracy, and enhance the quality of life for individuals living with this condition.

Importance of Adrenal Glands

The adrenal glands, two small glands located on top of your kidneys, play a vital role in maintaining your body's overall health and well-being. They are responsible for producing several essential hormones that regulate various bodily functions.

Key Hormones Produced by the Adrenal Glands:

- Cortisol: Often referred to as the "stress hormone," cortisol helps your body respond to stress, regulate blood sugar levels, and maintain blood pressure. It also plays a role in metabolism and immune function.
- Aldosterone: This hormone helps regulate the balance of sodium and potassium in your body, which is crucial for maintaining blood pressure and fluid balance.
- Adrenaline (epinephrine) and Noradrenaline (norepinephrine): These hormones, also known as catecholamines, prepare your body for the "fight-or-flight" response. They increase heart rate, blood pressure, and blood sugar levels, providing the energy needed to respond to danger or stress.

Importance of Adrenal Glands:

The adrenal glands are essential for several reasons:

- Stress Response: They help your body cope with stress by releasing cortisol, which helps regulate your body's response to various stressors, such as physical exertion, emotional distress, or illness.
- Blood Pressure Regulation: The adrenal glands produce aldosterone, which helps maintain blood pressure by regulating the balance of sodium and potassium in the body.
- Blood Sugar Regulation: Cortisol helps regulate blood sugar levels by increasing the production of glucose in the liver and reducing the uptake of glucose by cells.
- Immune Function: Cortisol plays a role in regulating the immune system, helping to balance the body's inflammatory response.
- Sexual Function: The adrenal glands produce small amounts of sex hormones, such as androgens, which contribute to the development of secondary sex characteristics and libido.

If the adrenal glands are not functioning properly, it can lead to a variety of health problems, including adrenal insufficiency, a condition in which the body does not produce enough cortisol.

Book Objectives and Scope

This book typically aim to provide comprehensive information about adrenal insufficiency, including its causes, symptoms, diagnosis, and treatment. The scope of these books often covers the following key areas:

Objectives of this book:

- Educate: This book aims to educate readers about adrenal insufficiency, providing clear and concise information about the condition, its causes, symptoms, diagnosis, and treatment.
- Inform: This book seeks to inform readers about the specific roles of the adrenal glands and the hormones they produce, such as cortisol and aldosterone.
- Empower: This book empowers readers by providing them with the knowledge and tools to manage their condition effectively,

including information on medication adherence, stress management, and emergency preparedness.

Scope of this book:

- Pathophysiology: This book delves into the complex mechanisms underlying adrenal insufficiency, exploring how the dysfunction of the adrenal glands can impact various bodily systems.
- Clinical Presentation: This book provides a comprehensive overview of the diverse range of symptoms associated with adrenal insufficiency, from subtle to severe, and discusses how these symptoms can vary between individuals.
- Diagnosis: This book explores the diagnostic process for adrenal insufficiency, including the role of medical history, physical examination, laboratory tests, and imaging studies.
- Treatment: This book offers detailed information on the various treatment options available for adrenal insufficiency, including hormone replacement therapy with corticosteroids and mineralocorticoids, and

discusses the importance of individualized treatment plans.

- Management: This book provides practical guidance on managing adrenal insufficiency, including tips on diet, exercise, stress management, and travel considerations.
- Complications: This book addresses the potential complications of adrenal insufficiency, such as adrenal crisis, and provides strategies for prevention and management.
- Quality of Life: This book explores the impact of adrenal insufficiency on quality of life and offers strategies for improving well-being, including coping mechanisms, support groups, and psychological counseling.

Target Audience

This book is primarily intended for individuals who have been diagnosed with adrenal insufficiency. It is designed to provide them with a comprehensive understanding of their condition and empower them to manage it effectively.

Additionally, this book can be a valuable resource for:

- Caregivers: Family members, friends, or professional caregivers who support individuals with adrenal insufficiency can benefit from understanding the condition and its management.
- Healthcare Professionals: Healthcare providers, including endocrinologists, primary care physicians, and nurses, can use this book as a reference to stay updated on the latest information regarding adrenal insufficiency.
- Medical Students and Residents: This book can be a valuable resource for medical students and residents who are interested in learning more about endocrine disorders and adrenal insufficiency in particular.

By providing clear and concise information, this book aims to improve the quality of life for individuals with adrenal insufficiency and their caregivers.

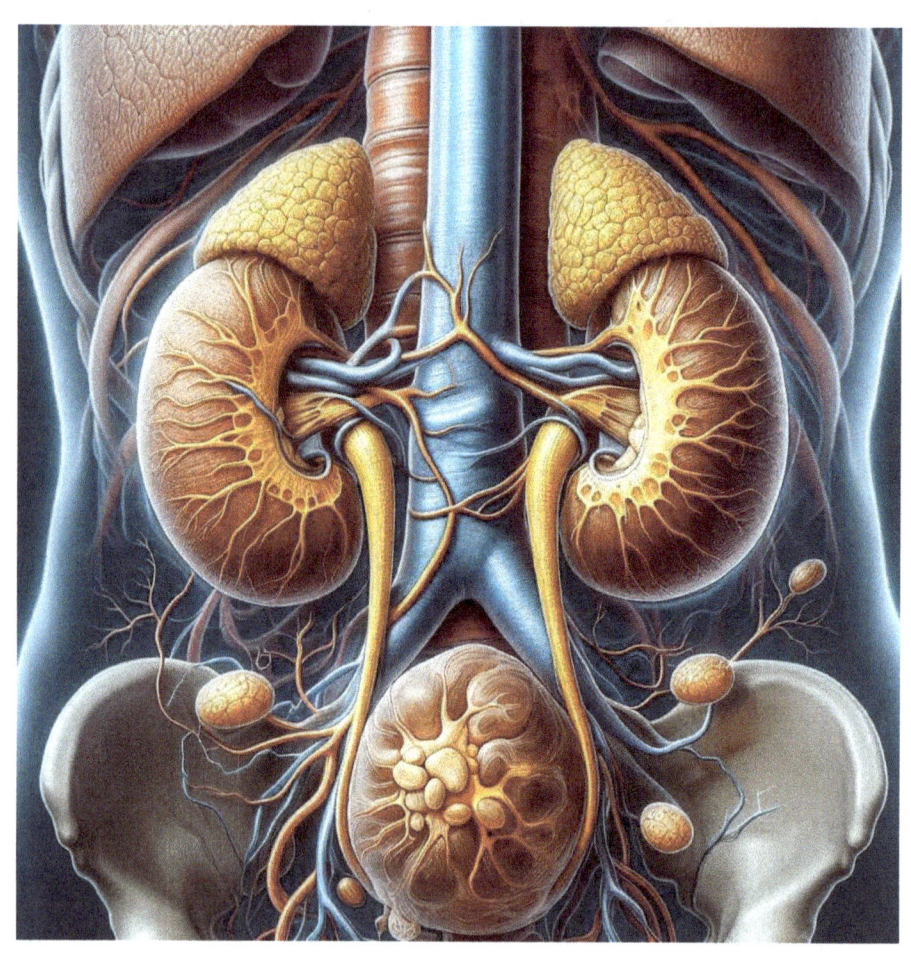

Part 2: Anatomy and Physiology

Adrenal Gland Anatomy

Location

The adrenal glands are two small, triangular-shaped glands that sit on top of your kidneys. They are about the size and shape of your thumb.

Structure

Each adrenal gland has two main parts:

- Adrenal Cortex: This is the outer layer of the gland. It is made up of three zones:

    - Zona Glomerulosa: This zone produces hormones called mineralocorticoids, which help regulate your body's salt and water balance.
    - Zona Fasciculata: This zone produces hormones called glucocorticoids, which help regulate your body's response to stress and inflammation.

- ○ Zona Reticularis: This zone produces hormones called androgens, which are male sex hormones.
- Adrenal Medulla: This is the inner layer of the gland. It produces hormones called catecholamines, which include adrenaline (epinephrine) and noradrenaline (norepinephrine). These hormones help your body respond to stress by increasing your heart rate, blood pressure, and blood sugar levels.

Blood Supply

The adrenal glands receive blood from several different arteries, including the superior adrenal artery, the middle adrenal artery, and the inferior adrenal artery. The blood is then drained from the adrenal glands by the adrenal veins, which empty into the inferior vena cava.

Nerve Supply

The adrenal glands are innervated by the sympathetic nervous system. This system helps to regulate the release of hormones from the adrenal medulla in response to stress.

Functions

The adrenal glands play an important role in many different bodily functions, including:

- Regulating blood pressure
- Regulating blood sugar levels
- Regulating the body's response to stress
- Regulating the body's salt and water balance
- Promoting growth and development
- Regulating the immune system

Hormones Produced by Adrenal Glands

The adrenal glands produce a variety of hormones that play crucial roles in regulating various bodily functions. Here's a breakdown of these hormones:

Hormones Produced by the Adrenal Cortex:

1. Mineralocorticoids (primarily Aldosterone):

    - Regulates electrolyte balance, particularly sodium and potassium levels in the blood.
    - Influences blood pressure by controlling water retention.

2. Glucocorticoids (primarily Cortisol):

    - Regulates the body's stress response.
    - Helps maintain blood sugar levels.
    - Suppresses inflammation.
    - Affects metabolism of proteins, carbohydrates, and fats.

3. Androgens (primarily DHEA):

    - Contribute to sexual development and function.
    - Influence muscle mass and bone density.
    - Play a role in libido and energy levels.

Hormones Produced by the Adrenal Medulla:

1. Catecholamines (Adrenaline and Noradrenaline):

- Prepare the body for the "fight-or-flight" response.
- Increase heart rate and blood pressure.
- Dilate airways for increased oxygen intake.
- Divert blood flow to vital organs.
- Increase blood sugar levels for energy.

It's important to note that the production and release of these hormones are carefully regulated by the hypothalamus and pituitary gland, forming a complex hormonal feedback system. Any imbalances in adrenal hormone production can lead to various health conditions, such as Cushing's syndrome, Addison's disease, or pheochromocytoma.

Regulation of Adrenal Function

The regulation of adrenal function is a complex interplay of hormonal signals and neural inputs. Here's a simplified overview:

Hypothalamic-Pituitary-Adrenal (HPA) Axis:

This axis is the primary regulator of adrenal cortex function. It involves three main components:

1. Hypothalamus:

    - Releases Corticotropin-Releasing Hormone (CRH) in response to stress, low blood sugar, or circadian rhythms.

2. Pituitary Gland:

    - CRH stimulates the pituitary to release Adrenocorticotropic Hormone (ACTH).
    - ACTH travels through the bloodstream to the adrenal cortex.
    -

3. Adrenal Cortex:

    - ACTH stimulates the adrenal cortex to produce cortisol and other glucocorticoids.
    - Cortisol levels rise, helping the body respond to stress.

Negative Feedback Loop:

- As cortisol levels increase, they signal the hypothalamus and pituitary to reduce CRH and ACTH production.
- This negative feedback loop helps maintain cortisol levels within a normal range.

Neural Regulation:

- The sympathetic nervous system, particularly during stress, directly stimulates the adrenal medulla to release adrenaline and noradrenaline.
- These hormones rapidly prepare the body for the "fight-or-flight" response.

Circadian Rhythm:

- The HPA axis is influenced by the body's internal clock.
- Cortisol levels naturally rise in the morning and decline in the evening.
- Disruptions to this circadian rhythm can affect adrenal function and overall health.

Factors Affecting Adrenal Function:

- Stress: Physical, emotional, or psychological stress can trigger the HPA axis.
- Sleep: Inadequate sleep can disrupt the HPA axis and lead to cortisol imbalances.
- Diet and Nutrition: Poor nutrition can affect adrenal function.
- Medications: Certain medications can interfere with adrenal hormone production.
- Underlying Medical Conditions: Diseases like adrenal insufficiency or Cushing's syndrome can affect adrenal function.

Adrenal Gland Disorders

Adrenal gland disorders can disrupt the delicate balance of hormones produced by these glands, leading to a variety of health issues. Here are some common adrenal gland disorders:

Hypercortisolism (Cushing's Syndrome):

- Cushing's Disease: This occurs when the pituitary gland produces excess ACTH, stimulating the adrenal glands to produce too much cortisol. Symptoms include weight gain, particularly in the face and abdomen, high blood pressure, muscle weakness, and skin thinning.
- Adrenal Cushing's Syndrome: This occurs when a tumor in the adrenal gland produces excess cortisol independently of pituitary control. Symptoms are similar to Cushing's disease.

Hyperaldosteronism (Conn's Syndrome):

- This condition occurs when the adrenal glands produce too much aldosterone, leading to high blood pressure, low potassium levels, and muscle weakness.

Pheochromocytoma:

- This is a rare tumor of the adrenal medulla that produces excess adrenaline and noradrenaline. Symptoms include sudden surges in blood pressure, rapid heart rate, sweating, headaches, and anxiety attacks.

Adrenal Cancer:

- Adrenal cancer is a rare type of cancer that can affect either the adrenal cortex or medulla. Symptoms may include abdominal pain, weight loss, fatigue, and hormonal imbalances.

Physiological Effects of Adrenal Hormones

The adrenal glands produce a variety of hormones that play crucial roles in regulating many bodily functions. Here's a breakdown of the physiological effects of these hormones:

Adrenal Cortex Hormones

1. Mineralocorticoids (primarily Aldosterone):
    - Electrolyte Balance: Regulates sodium and potassium levels in the blood.

- Blood Pressure: Influences blood pressure by controlling water retention.
- Renal Function: Affects kidney function by controlling sodium reabsorption.

2. Glucocorticoids (primarily Cortisol):

- Stress Response: Helps the body respond to stress by increasing blood sugar levels, suppressing inflammation, and mobilizing energy stores.
- Immune System: Suppresses the immune system.
- Metabolism: Affects the metabolism of carbohydrates, proteins, and fats.
- Blood Pressure: Can contribute to increased blood pressure.

3. Androgens (primarily DHEA):

- Sexual Development: Contributes to the development of secondary sex characteristics in both males and females.
- Libido: Influences libido and sexual function.

- Muscle Mass and Bone Density: Supports muscle mass and bone density.

Adrenal Medulla Hormones

1. Catecholamines (Adrenaline and Noradrenaline):
    - Heart Rate and Blood Pressure: Increases heart rate and blood pressure.
    - Blood Flow: Redistributes blood flow to vital organs (heart, brain, muscles).
    - Respiratory System: Dilates airways to increase oxygen intake.
    - Metabolism: Stimulates the breakdown of glycogen into glucose for energy.
    - Pupil Dilation: Dilates pupils to improve vision.
    - Sweating: Increases sweating to cool the body.
    - Mental Alertness: Enhances mental alertness and focus.

These hormones work together to maintain homeostasis and help the body adapt to various stressors.

Part 3: Types of Adrenal Insufficiency

Primary Adrenal Insufficiency (Addison's Disease)

Primary adrenal insufficiency, also known as Addison's disease, is a rare condition where your adrenal glands don't produce enough of the hormones cortisol and aldosterone. These hormones play crucial roles in your body's response to stress, blood pressure regulation, and electrolyte balance.

Causes

- Autoimmune: This is the most common cause, where your immune system mistakenly attacks your adrenal glands.
- Infections: Infections like tuberculosis or fungal infections can damage the adrenal glands.
- Hemorrhage: Bleeding into the adrenal glands can disrupt their function.

- Cancer: Cancer that spreads to the adrenal glands can affect their hormone production.
- Inherited Conditions: Some rare genetic disorders can lead to adrenal insufficiency.

Symptoms

Symptoms can develop gradually and may vary in severity:

- Fatigue and Weakness: You may feel persistently tired and weak, even after rest.
- Weight Loss: Unexplained weight loss can occur despite a normal appetite.
- Muscle Weakness: Difficulty with activities requiring muscle strength.
- Skin Changes: Darkening of the skin, especially in areas of creases like elbows and knees.
- Low Blood Pressure: You may experience dizziness or lightheadedness, especially when standing up.
- Salt Cravings: A desire for salty foods due to low sodium levels.

- Nausea, Vomiting, and Diarrhea: These symptoms can be severe, especially during an adrenal crisis.
- Depression and Mood Changes: Emotional disturbances can be associated with adrenal insufficiency.

Diagnosis

Diagnosis involves a combination of:

- Medical History and Physical Exam: Your doctor will ask about your symptoms and perform a physical examination.
- Blood Tests: To measure cortisol and aldosterone levels.
- Stimulation Tests: To assess your adrenal glands' response to stress.
- Imaging Tests: Such as CT scans or MRI to look for abnormalities in the adrenal glands.

Treatment

Treatment focuses on replacing the missing hormones:

- Hormone Replacement Therapy: You'll need to take medications containing cortisol and aldosterone, usually in pill form. The dosage will be adjusted based on your individual needs.
- Stress Management: During times of increased stress, such as illness or surgery, you may need additional hormone supplementation.
- Monitoring: Regular check-ups with your doctor are essential to monitor your hormone levels and adjust your medication as needed.

Secondary Adrenal Insufficiency

Secondary adrenal insufficiency is a condition where your adrenal glands don't produce enough cortisol because your pituitary gland isn't signaling them to do so. The pituitary gland, located at the base of your brain, produces a hormone called adrenocorticotropic hormone (ACTH), which stimulates the adrenal glands to produce cortisol.

Causes

- Pituitary Gland Disorders: Conditions like pituitary tumors or infections can damage the pituitary gland and reduce ACTH production.
- Medications: Certain medications, such as corticosteroids (like prednisone), can suppress the natural production of cortisol by your adrenal glands. When these medications are stopped abruptly, it can take time for your adrenal glands to resume normal function.
- Other Medical Conditions: Some chronic illnesses, such as tuberculosis or HIV, can affect the pituitary gland and lead to secondary adrenal insufficiency.

Symptoms

Symptoms of secondary adrenal insufficiency are similar to those of primary adrenal insufficiency, but they may develop more gradually:

- Fatigue and Weakness: Persistent tiredness and lack of energy.

- Muscle Weakness: Difficulty with activities requiring muscle strength.
- Joint and Muscle Pain: Aches and pains in your joints and muscles.
- Weight Loss: Unexplained weight loss, even with a normal appetite.
- Low Blood Pressure: Dizziness or lightheadedness, especially when standing up.
- Nausea, Vomiting, and Loss of Appetite: Digestive issues.
- Depression and Mood Changes: Emotional disturbances.

Diagnosis

Diagnosis involves a combination of:

- Medical History and Physical Exam: Your doctor will ask about your symptoms and perform a physical examination.
- Blood Tests: To measure cortisol and ACTH levels.
- Stimulation Tests: To assess your adrenal glands' response to ACTH.

- Imaging Tests: Such as MRI or CT scans to evaluate the pituitary gland.

Treatment

Treatment focuses on addressing the underlying cause and replacing the missing cortisol:

- Treating the Underlying Cause: If a specific condition is causing the secondary adrenal insufficiency, treatment will focus on managing that condition.
- Hormone Replacement Therapy: You'll need to take medication containing cortisol, usually in pill form. The dosage will be adjusted based on your individual needs.
- Stress Management: During times of increased stress, such as illness or surgery, you may need additional hormone supplementation.
- Monitoring: Regular check-ups with your doctor are essential to monitor your hormone levels and adjust your medication as needed.

Tertiary Adrenal Insufficiency

Tertiary adrenal insufficiency is a less common condition where your adrenal glands fail to respond to ACTH, even though your pituitary gland is producing normal levels of it. This can occur due to prolonged exposure to high levels of cortisol, such as during long-term corticosteroid therapy.

Causes

- Long-term Corticosteroid Use: Prolonged use of corticosteroids can suppress the natural production of cortisol by your adrenal glands. When these medications are stopped abruptly, it can take time for your adrenal glands to resume normal function.
- Other Medical Conditions: Some rare medical conditions, such as certain infections or autoimmune disorders, can directly affect the adrenal glands and impair their response to ACTH.

Symptoms

Symptoms of tertiary adrenal insufficiency are similar to those of primary and secondary adrenal insufficiency:

- Fatigue and Weakness: Persistent tiredness and lack of energy.
- Muscle Weakness: Difficulty with activities requiring muscle strength.
- Joint and Muscle Pain: Aches and pains in your joints and muscles.
- Weight Loss: Unexplained weight loss, even with a normal appetite.
- Low Blood Pressure: Dizziness or lightheadedness, especially when standing up.
- Nausea, Vomiting, and Loss of Appetite: Digestive issues.
- Depression and Mood Changes: Emotional disturbances.

Diagnosis

Diagnosis involves a combination of:

- Medical History and Physical Exam: Your doctor will ask about your symptoms and perform a physical examination.
- Blood Tests: To measure cortisol and ACTH levels.
- Stimulation Tests: To assess your adrenal glands' response to ACTH.
- Imaging Tests: Such as MRI or CT scans to evaluate the pituitary gland and adrenal glands.

Treatment

Treatment focuses on:

- Gradual Withdrawal of Corticosteroids: If you're taking corticosteroids, your doctor will gradually reduce the dosage to allow your adrenal glands to regain function.
- Hormone Replacement Therapy: In some cases, you may need to take medication containing cortisol, especially during periods of stress or illness.

- Monitoring: Regular check-ups with your doctor are essential to monitor your hormone levels and adjust your treatment as needed.

It's important to note that if you're taking corticosteroids, you should never stop taking them abruptly without consulting your doctor. Sudden withdrawal can lead to an adrenal crisis, a life-threatening condition.

Congenital Adrenal Hyperplasia (CAH)

Congenital Adrenal Hyperplasia (CAH) is a rare genetic disorder that affects the adrenal glands. These glands are located on top of your kidneys and produce various hormones, including cortisol and aldosterone. In CAH, the adrenal glands don't produce enough cortisol, and in some cases, also produce excessive amounts of male hormones (androgens).

Types of CAH

There are different types of CAH, classified based on the specific enzyme deficiency:

- Classic CAH: The most common type, characterized by severe cortisol deficiency and excess androgen production.
- Non-classic CAH: A milder form with less severe cortisol deficiency and androgen excess.

Causes

CAH is caused by genetic mutations that affect the enzymes involved in cortisol production. These genetic mutations are usually inherited from parents who carry the defective gene.

Symptoms

Symptoms of CAH vary depending on the type and severity of the condition:

In Females:

- Ambiguous Genitalia: At birth, the external genitalia may appear masculine due to excess androgen exposure.

- Early Puberty: Early development of pubic hair, body hair, and breast buds.
- Irregular Menstrual Cycles: Irregular or absent periods.
- Infertility: Difficulty conceiving due to hormonal imbalances.
- Excess Hair Growth: Excessive hair growth on the face, chest, and back.
- Acne: Severe acne.

In Males:

- Rapid Growth: Accelerated growth during childhood.
- Early Puberty: Early development of pubic hair and body hair.
- Advanced Bone Age: Bones may mature faster than expected.
- Behavioral Issues: Some children with CAH may exhibit behavioral problems, such as aggression or hyperactivity.

Diagnosis

Diagnosis of CAH involves:

- Physical Examination: A thorough physical examination to assess physical development and any abnormalities.
- Hormone Tests: Blood tests to measure cortisol, ACTH, and androgen levels.
- Genetic Testing: To identify the specific genetic mutation causing CAH.

Treatment

Treatment for CAH aims to:

- Replace Cortisol: Hormone replacement therapy with cortisol medication to regulate hormone levels and prevent adrenal crises.
- Manage Androgen Excess: In some cases, medications may be used to block the effects of excess androgens.
- Surgical Correction: For females with ambiguous genitalia, surgery may be necessary to correct the appearance of the genitals.
- Psychological Support: Counseling and support for individuals with CAH and their families.

With proper treatment, individuals with CAH can lead normal and healthy lives. Regular medical follow-up is essential to monitor hormone levels and adjust treatment as needed.

Adrenal Crisis

An adrenal crisis is a life-threatening condition that occurs when your body doesn't produce enough cortisol, a hormone essential for regulating stress response, blood pressure, and blood sugar levels. It can happen in people with adrenal insufficiency, a condition where the adrenal glands don't produce enough hormones, or in those who suddenly stop taking corticosteroids.

Causes of Adrenal Crisis

- Untreated Adrenal Insufficiency: If you have adrenal insufficiency and aren't receiving proper treatment, you're at risk of an adrenal crisis.

- Sudden Withdrawal of Corticosteroids: Abruptly stopping corticosteroids, even if you've been taking them for a long time, can trigger an adrenal crisis.
- Stressful Events: Physical or emotional stress, such as illness, surgery, or trauma, can increase the body's demand for cortisol and may lead to a crisis.
- Infection: Infections can worsen adrenal insufficiency and increase the risk of a crisis.

Symptoms of Adrenal Crisis

Symptoms of an adrenal crisis can develop rapidly and can be severe:

- Severe Fatigue and Weakness: Extreme tiredness and lack of energy.
- Severe Abdominal Pain: Intense pain in the abdomen.
- Vomiting and Diarrhea: Persistent nausea, vomiting, and diarrhea.
- Low Blood Pressure: Dizziness, lightheadedness, or fainting.

- Rapid Heart Rate: A fast and irregular heartbeat.
- Dehydration: Dry mouth, decreased urine output, and dark urine.
- Confusion and Disorientation: Mental confusion and difficulty thinking clearly.
- Loss of Consciousness: In severe cases, individuals may lose consciousness.

Diagnosis

If you experience symptoms of an adrenal crisis, it's crucial to seek immediate medical attention. Your doctor will perform a physical examination and order blood tests to measure cortisol levels.

Treatment

Treatment for an adrenal crisis is aimed at restoring cortisol levels and stabilizing vital signs:

- Intravenous Fluids: To treat dehydration and maintain blood pressure.
- Hydrocortisone: A synthetic form of cortisol administered intravenously to quickly replace the missing hormone.

- Electrolyte Replacement: To correct imbalances in sodium, potassium, and other electrolytes.
- Monitoring: Close monitoring of vital signs, blood sugar levels, and electrolyte levels.

Prevention

To prevent adrenal crises, it's important to:

- Adhere to Treatment: If you have adrenal insufficiency, follow your doctor's treatment plan and take your medications as prescribed.
- Carry Emergency Medication: Carry a self-injectable form of hydrocortisone, such as a pre-filled syringe, in case of a crisis.
- Wear a Medical Alert Bracelet or Necklace: Inform others about your condition and the need for emergency treatment.
- Avoid Stressful Situations: If possible, avoid situations that may trigger a crisis, such as severe illness or injury.
- Inform Healthcare Providers: Always inform your healthcare providers about your

condition, especially before any medical procedures or surgeries.

By taking these precautions and seeking prompt medical attention, you can reduce the risk of an adrenal crisis and manage your condition effectively.

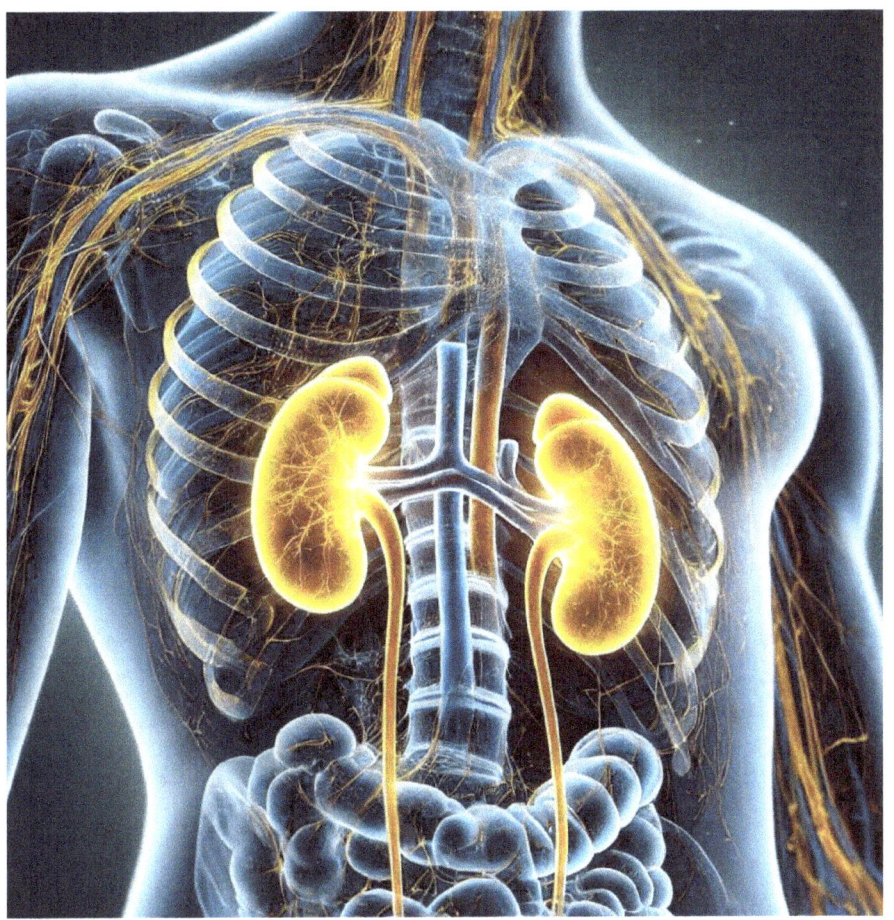

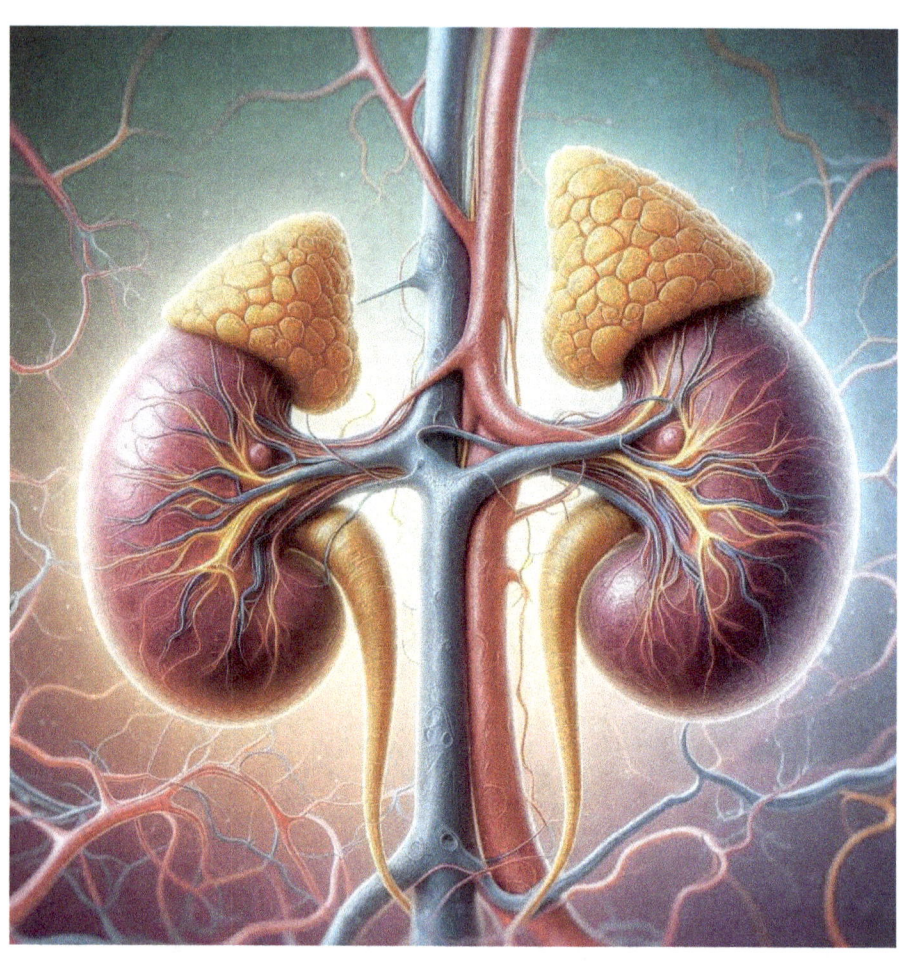

Part 4: Causes and Risk Factors

Genetic Causes

Let's delve into the specific genetic conditions that can lead to this health issue.

Congenital Adrenal Hyperplasia (CAH)

CAH is a group of genetic disorders that affect the adrenal glands' ability to produce hormones like cortisol and aldosterone. These glands are located on top of your kidneys and play a crucial role in managing stress, blood pressure, and electrolyte balance. In CAH, a missing or faulty enzyme disrupts the normal hormone production process.

Familial Glucocorticoid Deficiency (FGD)

FGD is a rare genetic condition that impairs the production of cortisol. This can lead to adrenal insufficiency and other related symptoms. FGD is often inherited in an autosomal recessive pattern, meaning that both parents must carry a copy of the faulty gene for their child to be affected.

Autoimmune Adrenalitis

While not directly genetic, autoimmune adrenalitis is a condition where your body's immune system mistakenly attacks and damages the adrenal glands. It's believed that genetic factors can make some people more susceptible to developing this autoimmune disorder.

Other Genetic Syndromes

Several other genetic syndromes can include adrenal insufficiency as one of their symptoms. These syndromes often involve multiple organ systems and can have a wide range of associated features. Some examples include:

- Triple A Syndrome (Allgrove Syndrome): This rare disorder affects the autonomic nervous system, the adrenal glands, and the eyes.
- Smith-Lemli-Opitz Syndrome: This syndrome affects cholesterol production and can lead to adrenal insufficiency.
- Wolman Disease: This disorder affects lipid metabolism and can cause adrenal insufficiency.

Identifying Genetic Causes

If you or your child is diagnosed with adrenal insufficiency, your doctor may recommend genetic testing to determine the underlying cause. This can help guide treatment decisions and provide information about the potential for passing the condition on to future generations.

Autoimmune Disorders

What are Autoimmune Disorders?

Autoimmune disorders occur when your body's immune system, which is designed to protect you from invaders like bacteria and viruses, mistakenly attacks your own tissues. This can lead to a range of health problems, including adrenal insufficiency.

Autoimmune Adrenalitis

Autoimmune adrenalitis is the most common autoimmune cause of adrenal insufficiency. In this condition, your immune system targets and damages the adrenal glands, leading to reduced hormone production.

Type 1 Diabetes

Type 1 diabetes is an autoimmune disease that affects the pancreas, specifically the cells that produce insulin. While it primarily affects blood sugar control, it can also increase the risk of developing other autoimmune conditions, including adrenal insufficiency. This association is thought to be due to shared genetic and environmental factors that predispose individuals to autoimmune diseases.

Hashimoto's Thyroiditis

Hashimoto's thyroiditis is another autoimmune disorder that targets the thyroid gland. It can lead to underactive thyroid function (hypothyroidism). While not directly causing adrenal insufficiency, it can increase the risk of developing other autoimmune conditions, including autoimmune adrenalitis.

Other Autoimmune Disorders

Several other autoimmune disorders have been linked to an increased risk of adrenal insufficiency, including:

- Rheumatoid arthritis
- Systemic lupus erythematosus (SLE)
- Graves' disease
- Celiac disease
- Vitiligo

Identifying Autoimmune Causes

If you or your doctor suspect that your adrenal insufficiency is caused by an autoimmune disorder, several tests may be performed to confirm the diagnosis. These tests may include:

- Blood tests: To measure hormone levels and look for signs of autoimmune activity.
- Autoantibody testing: To identify specific antibodies that target the adrenal glands.
- Imaging tests: To assess the size and function of the adrenal glands.

Infections

Tuberculosis (TB)

Tuberculosis, a bacterial infection primarily affecting the lungs, can sometimes spread to other organs, including the adrenal glands. This can lead to adrenal tuberculosis, a rare but serious condition that can cause adrenal insufficiency.

Fungal Infections

Fungal infections, such as histoplasmosis and coccidioidomycosis, can also affect the adrenal glands. These infections, often contracted by inhaling fungal spores, can lead to adrenal inflammation and damage, resulting in adrenal insufficiency.

Viral Infections

While less common, certain viral infections can also contribute to adrenal insufficiency. For example, HIV infection can weaken the immune system, making individuals more susceptible to opportunistic infections, including those that can affect the adrenal glands. Additionally, some viruses, such as cytomegalovirus (CMV), can directly infect the adrenal glands and cause damage.

Parasitic Infections

Parasitic infections, such as those caused by the parasite *Trypanosoma cruzi* (which causes Chagas disease), can also affect the adrenal glands. These parasites can invade the adrenal tissue and cause inflammation and damage, leading to adrenal insufficiency.

Identifying Infectious Causes

If your doctor suspects that your adrenal insufficiency is caused by an infection, they may perform a variety of tests to confirm the diagnosis. These tests may include:

- Blood tests: To check for signs of infection and measure hormone levels.
- Imaging tests: Such as CT scans or MRIs, to assess the size and appearance of the adrenal glands.

- Microbiological tests: To identify the specific infectious agent, such as a culture or a blood test for antibodies.

Treatment and Management

Treatment for adrenal insufficiency caused by an infection depends on the specific type of infection and its severity. In many cases, treatment focuses on eradicating the infection with appropriate medications, such as antibiotics, antifungals, or antivirals. Once the infection is under control, hormone replacement therapy may be needed to manage adrenal insufficiency.

Trauma and Surgery

Adrenal insufficiency can also be triggered by various traumatic events, including surgeries and injuries. Let's delve into how these factors can lead to this health issue.

Adrenal Gland Injury

- Accidental Trauma: Direct trauma to the abdomen, such as in car accidents or falls, can injure the adrenal glands. This injury can disrupt their normal function and lead to temporary or permanent adrenal insufficiency.
- Penetrating Trauma: Gunshot wounds or stab wounds that directly penetrate the adrenal glands can cause significant damage and lead to adrenal insufficiency.

Adrenal Gland Surgery

- Adrenalectomy: Surgical removal of one or both adrenal glands, often performed to treat adrenal tumors or cancer, inevitably results in adrenal insufficiency. If only one gland is removed, the remaining gland may be able to compensate for some time, but eventually, hormone replacement therapy will be necessary.
- Other Surgeries: Surgeries in the abdominal region, such as kidney or liver transplants, can sometimes inadvertently damage the adrenal

glands, leading to temporary or permanent adrenal insufficiency.

Identifying Trauma-Related Adrenal Insufficiency

If your doctor suspects that your adrenal insufficiency is caused by trauma or surgery, they may perform a variety of tests to confirm the diagnosis. These tests may include:

- Blood tests: To measure hormone levels and assess adrenal function.
- Imaging tests: Such as CT scans or MRIs, to visualize the adrenal glands and assess any damage.

Medication and Substances

Corticosteroids

- Long-term Use: Prolonged use of high-dose corticosteroids, often prescribed for conditions like asthma, arthritis, or autoimmune diseases, can suppress the natural production of cortisol by the adrenal glands. When these medications are abruptly stopped, the adrenal glands may not be able to quickly resume normal function, leading to adrenal insufficiency.

- Sudden Withdrawal: Abruptly stopping long-term corticosteroid use can also trigger adrenal insufficiency. This is why it's crucial to taper off these medications gradually under the supervision of a healthcare provider.

Other Medications

- Antifungal Medications: Certain antifungal medications, such as ketoconazole, can interfere with the production of adrenal hormones.
- Chemotherapy Drugs: Some chemotherapy drugs can damage the adrenal glands, leading to temporary or permanent adrenal insufficiency.
- HIV Medications: Certain medications used to treat HIV infection can also affect adrenal function.

Alcohol

Excessive alcohol consumption can damage the liver, which plays a role in hormone metabolism. Liver damage can impair the body's ability to produce and use hormones, including those from the adrenal glands.

Other Substances

- Illicit Drugs: Some illicit drugs, such as cocaine and heroin, can directly damage the adrenal glands or indirectly affect their function through their impact on the immune system.
- Environmental Toxins: Exposure to certain environmental toxins, such as heavy metals, can also damage the adrenal glands and lead to adrenal insufficiency.

Identifying Medication-Induced Adrenal Insufficiency

If your doctor suspects that your adrenal insufficiency is caused by medication or substance use, they may perform a variety of tests to confirm the diagnosis. These tests may include:

- Blood tests: To measure hormone levels and assess adrenal function.
- Urine tests: To check for signs of adrenal insufficiency and to monitor medication levels.

Other Medical Conditions

Adrenal insufficiency can also be a secondary effect of various medical conditions. Let's delve into how these underlying health issues can lead to this complication.

Cancer

- Primary Adrenal Cancer: Cancer originating within the adrenal glands can directly damage the gland tissue, leading to adrenal insufficiency.
- Cancers Metastatic to the Adrenal Glands: Cancers from other parts of the body, such as lung, breast, or kidney cancer, can spread (metastasize) to the adrenal glands. These metastatic tumors can disrupt the normal

function of the adrenal glands, causing adrenal insufficiency.

- Cancer Treatments: Certain cancer treatments, such as chemotherapy and radiation therapy, can damage the adrenal glands as a side effect, leading to temporary or permanent adrenal insufficiency.

HIV Infection

HIV infection can weaken the immune system, making individuals more susceptible to opportunistic infections, including those that can affect the adrenal glands. Additionally, some HIV medications can directly impact adrenal function.

Liver Disease

The liver plays a crucial role in the metabolism of hormones. Severe liver disease can impair the liver's ability to process hormones, leading to hormonal imbalances, including adrenal insufficiency.

Kidney Disease

The kidneys play a role in regulating electrolyte balance, which is essential for proper adrenal gland function. Severe kidney disease can disrupt this balance, leading to adrenal insufficiency. Additionally, certain medications used to treat kidney disease, such as corticosteroids, can also contribute to adrenal insufficiency.

Identifying Secondary Adrenal Insufficiency

If your doctor suspects that your adrenal insufficiency is secondary to another medical condition, they may perform a variety of tests to confirm the diagnosis. These tests may include:

- Blood tests: To measure hormone levels and assess adrenal function.
- Imaging tests: Such as CT scans or MRIs, to visualize the adrenal glands and identify any underlying conditions.
- Other tests: Depending on the suspected underlying cause, additional tests may be necessary, such as liver function tests, kidney function tests, or tumor markers.

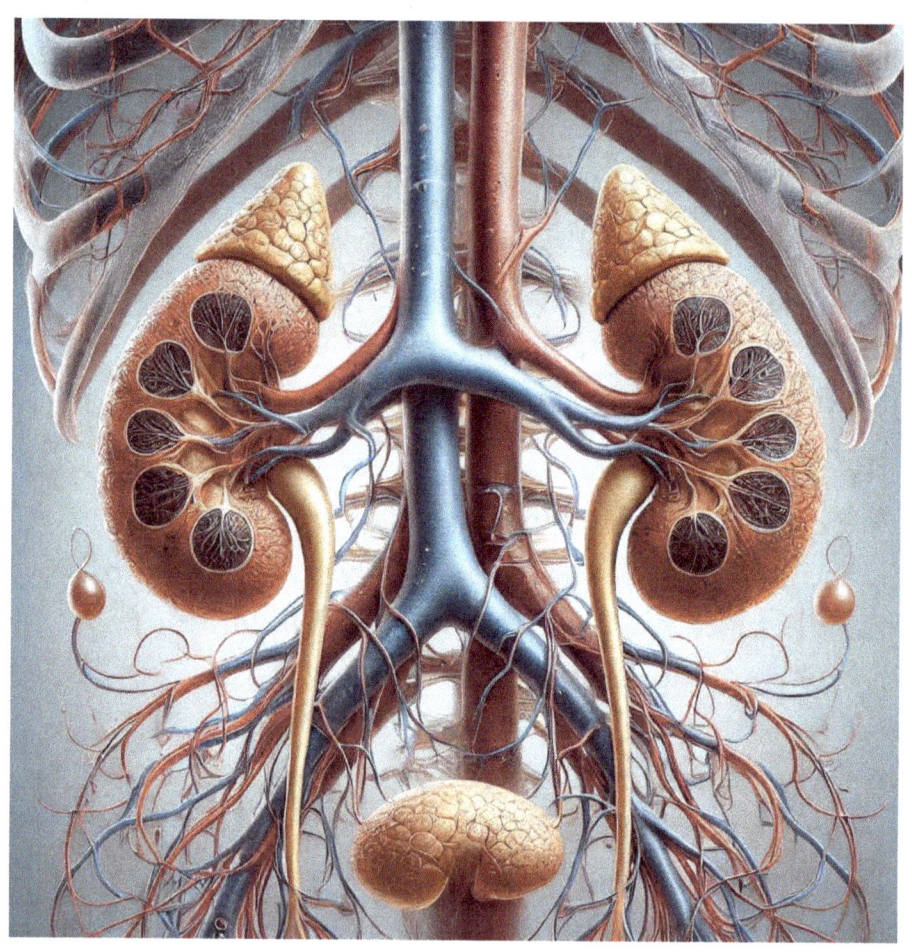

Part 5: Symptoms and Diagnosis

Clinical Presentation

The clinical presentation of adrenal insufficiency can vary depending on the severity and underlying cause. However, some common symptoms include:

Chronic Adrenal Insufficiency

- Fatigue: This is often the most prominent symptom, causing a feeling of persistent tiredness and exhaustion.
- Muscle Weakness: Difficulty performing daily activities and weakness in the muscles.
- Weight Loss: Unexplained weight loss despite a normal or increased appetite.
- Anorexia and Nausea: Loss of appetite and frequent feelings of nausea.
- Abdominal Pain: Vague abdominal discomfort or pain.
- Low Blood Pressure (Hypotension): This can lead to dizziness, lightheadedness, or fainting, especially when standing up from a sitting or lying position.

- Salt Craving: A strong desire for salty foods due to the body's need for sodium.
- Hyperpigmentation: Darkening of the skin, especially in areas exposed to sunlight or areas of friction, such as the elbows, knees, and knuckles. This is caused by increased production of melanin, a skin pigment.
- Menstrual Irregularities: Irregular or absent menstrual periods in women.
- Decreased Libido: Reduced sexual desire in both men and women.
- Depression and Irritability: Changes in mood, including irritability, depression, and difficulty concentrating.
- Hypoglycemia: Low blood sugar levels, which can cause symptoms like shakiness, sweating, and confusion.

Acute Adrenal Insufficiency (Adrenal Crisis)

Acute adrenal insufficiency, also known as an adrenal crisis, is a life-threatening condition that requires immediate medical attention. Symptoms can develop rapidly and include:

- Severe Fatigue and Weakness: Feeling extremely tired and weak, unable to perform even simple tasks.
- Severe Abdominal Pain: Intense pain in the abdomen.
- Severe Vomiting and Diarrhea: Persistent vomiting and diarrhea, leading to dehydration.
- Low Blood Pressure: Significantly low blood pressure, causing dizziness, fainting, and shock.
- Rapid Heart Rate (Tachycardia): Increased heart rate as the body tries to compensate for low blood pressure.
- Fever: Elevated body temperature.
- Confusion and Altered Mental Status: Difficulty thinking clearly, confusion, or even coma in severe cases.

Physical Examination

A physical examination is a crucial part of diagnosing adrenal insufficiency. During the exam, your doctor will look for specific signs and symptoms that may indicate the condition.

Here are some of the key findings that a doctor may look for:

General Appearance

- Fatigue and Weakness: Your doctor may observe that you appear tired, weak, and have difficulty with activities of daily living.
- Weight Loss: Unexplained weight loss, even if your appetite is normal or increased.
- Postural Hypotension: A drop in blood pressure when you stand up from a sitting or lying position. This can cause dizziness or lightheadedness.

Vital Signs

- Low Blood Pressure: Your blood pressure may be lower than normal, especially when you stand up.
- Rapid Heart Rate (Tachycardia): Your heart rate may be elevated, especially in response to stress or exertion.

Skin Examination

- Hyperpigmentation: Darkening of the skin, particularly in areas exposed to sunlight or areas of friction, such as the elbows, knees, and knuckles. This is caused by increased production of melanin, a skin pigment.
- Poor Wound Healing: Slow wound healing due to impaired tissue repair.

Abdominal Examination

- Abdominal Tenderness: Your doctor may feel tenderness in your abdomen, particularly in the adrenal gland region.

Neurological Examination

- Muscle Weakness: Your doctor may test your muscle strength to assess for weakness, especially in the proximal muscle groups (shoulders, hips, thighs).
- Reflexes: Your reflexes may be decreased or absent.

Other Examinations

- Oral Cavity: Your doctor may examine your oral cavity for signs of mucosal pigmentation.
- Genital Examination: In women, your doctor may examine your genitals for signs of decreased pubic hair or vulvar atrophy.

Laboratory Tests

To diagnose adrenal insufficiency, your doctor may order a series of laboratory tests. These tests help assess the function of your adrenal glands and identify any underlying causes of the condition.

Here are some of the common laboratory tests used to diagnose adrenal insufficiency:

Blood Tests

- Cortisol Level Tests:
    - Morning Cortisol Level: This test measures the level of cortisol in your blood early in the morning, typically between 6 AM and 8 AM. Low levels of cortisol at this time suggest adrenal insufficiency.
    - Cosyntropin Stimulation Test: This test involves administering a synthetic hormone called cosyntropin, which stimulates the adrenal glands to produce cortisol. Blood samples are taken before and after the injection to measure the cortisol response. A failure to increase cortisol levels in response to cosyntropin indicates adrenal insufficiency.
- Electrolyte Tests:
    - Sodium and Potassium Levels: Adrenal insufficiency can lead to imbalances in sodium and potassium levels in your

blood. Low sodium levels (hyponatremia) and high potassium levels (hyperkalemia) can be seen in this condition.

- Kidney Function Tests:
  - Blood Urea Nitrogen (BUN) and Creatinine: These tests assess kidney function. Adrenal insufficiency can sometimes affect kidney function, especially in severe cases.
- Autoantibody Tests:
  - Adrenal Autoantibodies: These tests can help identify autoimmune conditions that may be causing adrenal insufficiency. Autoimmune diseases, such as Addison's disease, involve the body's immune system attacking its own tissues, including the adrenal glands.
- Other Tests:
  - ACTH Level: This test measures the level of adrenocorticotropic hormone (ACTH), a hormone produced by the pituitary gland that stimulates the adrenal glands. In some cases of adrenal insufficiency, ACTH levels may be elevated.

- Insulin-Like Growth Factor-1 (IGF-1) Level: Low levels of IGF-1 can be seen in adrenal insufficiency, as it is a hormone regulated by cortisol.

Imaging Studies

- CT Scan or MRI: These imaging tests can help visualize the adrenal glands and identify any abnormalities, such as tumors or infections.

Specialized Tests

- 24-Hour Urine Cortisol Test: This test collects your urine over a 24-hour period to measure the total amount of cortisol excreted. Low levels of cortisol in the urine can indicate adrenal insufficiency.

It's important to note that the specific tests your doctor orders will depend on your individual symptoms and medical history. A combination of these tests is often necessary to make an accurate diagnosis of adrenal insufficiency.

Differential Diagnosis

Adrenal insufficiency can present with a wide range of symptoms, some of which may overlap with other conditions. A differential diagnosis is a process of identifying the most likely diagnosis from a list of possible conditions.

Here are some conditions that may mimic the symptoms of adrenal insufficiency and should be considered in the differential diagnosis:

Endocrine Disorders

- Hypothyroidism: This condition, caused by underactive thyroid gland, can lead to fatigue, weight gain, and muscle weakness.
- Diabetes Mellitus: Low blood sugar (hypoglycemia) can mimic some symptoms of adrenal insufficiency.
- Pituitary Disorders: Conditions affecting the pituitary gland, such as hypopituitarism, can lead to hormonal deficiencies, including adrenal insufficiency.

Non-Endocrine Disorders

- Chronic Fatigue Syndrome: This condition can cause persistent fatigue, muscle pain, and cognitive difficulties.
- Depression: Symptoms of depression, such as fatigue, loss of appetite, and difficulty concentrating, can be similar to those of adrenal insufficiency.
- Chronic Infections: Chronic infections, such as tuberculosis or HIV, can affect adrenal gland function.
- Malnutrition: Inadequate intake of nutrients can lead to hormonal imbalances and weakness.
- Certain Medications: Some medications, such as corticosteroids, can suppress adrenal gland function if abruptly stopped.

It's important to note that a comprehensive medical history, physical examination, and laboratory tests are essential to differentiate adrenal insufficiency from other conditions. A healthcare provider will carefully evaluate the patient's symptoms, medical history, and test results to arrive at an accurate diagnosis.

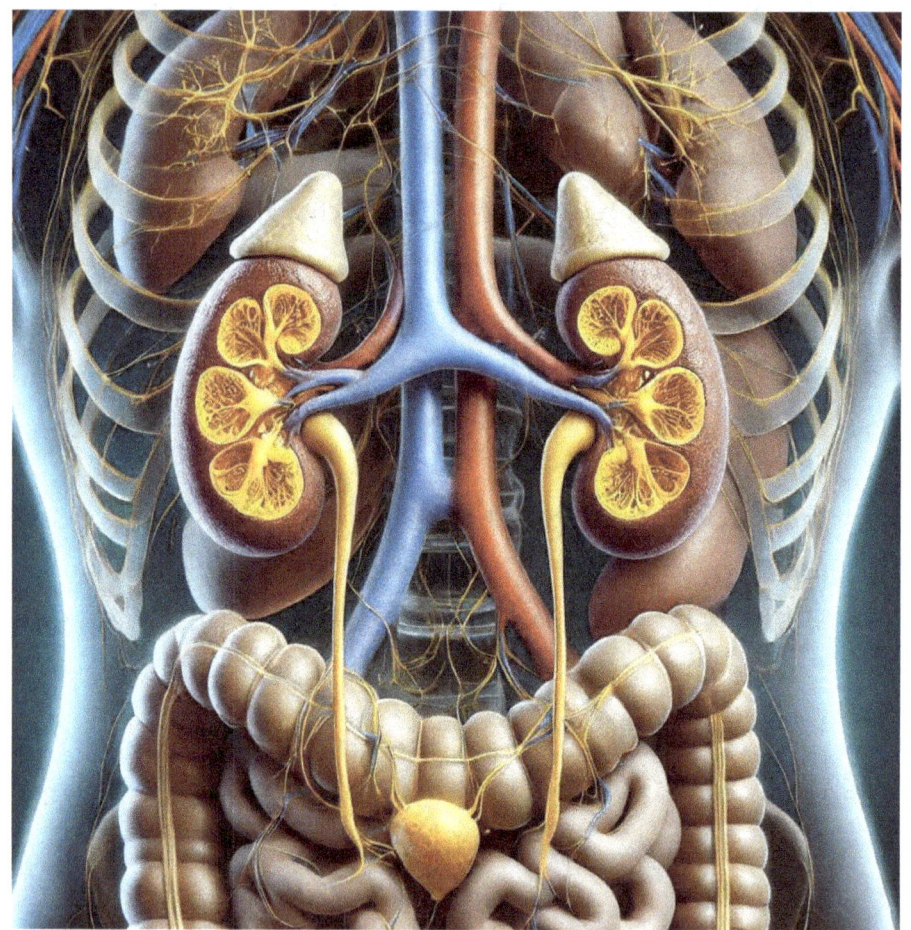

Part 6: Treatment and Management

Glucocorticoid Replacement Therapy

Glucocorticoid replacement therapy is a vital treatment for adrenal insufficiency, a condition where your adrenal glands don't produce enough hormones. This therapy aims to replace the hormones your body would normally produce, helping you maintain normal bodily functions.

Types of Glucocorticoids:

The most commonly used glucocorticoid for replacement therapy is hydrocortisone. It closely mimics the natural cortisol hormone produced by your adrenal glands. Other glucocorticoids like prednisone or prednisolone can also be used, but they have a different potency and duration of action compared to hydrocortisone.

Dosages:

The dosage of glucocorticoid replacement therapy is tailored to each individual's needs. It's determined by factors like your age, weight, overall health, and the severity of your adrenal insufficiency. Your doctor will carefully monitor your progress and adjust your dosage as needed.

Monitoring:

Regular monitoring is crucial to ensure your glucocorticoid replacement therapy is working effectively and safely. This typically involves:

- Blood tests: These tests measure your cortisol levels, electrolyte levels (like sodium and potassium), and kidney function. They help assess your adrenal function and identify any imbalances.
- Urine tests: Urine tests can measure cortisol levels and help monitor your overall adrenal function.
- Physical exams: Your doctor will perform regular physical exams to check for signs of adrenal insufficiency, such as fatigue, weakness, low blood pressure, and changes in skin pigmentation.

Adjustments:

Your glucocorticoid replacement therapy may need adjustments over time due to various factors:

- Changes in your health: If you develop other health conditions or experience significant stress, your dosage may need to be temporarily increased.
- Medication interactions: Some medications can interact with glucocorticoids, affecting their absorption or metabolism. Your doctor may need to adjust your dosage or consider alternative medications.
- Lifestyle changes: Major lifestyle changes, such as pregnancy, surgery, or significant illness, may require temporary dosage adjustments to cope with increased stress on your body.

Important Considerations:

- Stress dosing: If you experience significant physical or emotional stress, you may need to temporarily increase your glucocorticoid dosage to help your body cope. This is known as "stress dosing" and is essential to prevent adrenal crisis, a life-threatening condition.

- Injections: In some cases, your doctor may recommend injectable glucocorticoids, such as hydrocortisone injections, for emergencies or during periods of severe stress.
- Mineralocorticoid replacement: In addition to glucocorticoid replacement, you may also need mineralocorticoid replacement therapy, such as fludrocortisone, to regulate salt and water balance in your body.

By understanding the types of glucocorticoids, appropriate dosages, monitoring strategies, and potential adjustments, you can work closely with your doctor to optimize your glucocorticoid replacement therapy and manage your adrenal insufficiency effectively.

Mineralocorticoid Replacement Therapy

Mineralocorticoid replacement therapy is a crucial component of managing adrenal insufficiency, a condition where your adrenal glands don't produce enough hormones. This therapy aims to replace the mineralocorticoid hormone aldosterone, which helps regulate salt and water balance in your body.

Types of Mineralocorticoids:

The most commonly used mineralocorticoid for replacement therapy is fludrocortisone. It closely mimics the natural aldosterone hormone produced by your adrenal glands.

Dosages:

The dosage of mineralocorticoid replacement therapy is carefully determined by your doctor based on your individual needs. It's influenced by factors such as your age, weight, overall health, and the severity of your adrenal insufficiency. Your doctor will monitor your progress and adjust your dosage as needed.

Monitoring:

Regular monitoring is essential to ensure that your mineralocorticoid replacement therapy is working effectively and safely. This typically involves:

- Blood tests: These tests measure your electrolyte levels, particularly sodium and potassium, to assess your salt and water balance.
- Blood pressure monitoring: Regular blood pressure checks help monitor your cardiovascular health and ensure that your blood pressure is within a healthy range.

Adjustments:

Your mineralocorticoid replacement therapy may require adjustments over time due to various factors:

- Changes in your health: If you develop other health conditions or experience significant stress, your dosage may need to be temporarily increased.
- Medication interactions: Some medications can interact with mineralocorticoids, affecting their absorption or metabolism. Your doctor may need to adjust your dosage or consider alternative medications.

- Lifestyle changes: Major lifestyle changes, such as pregnancy, surgery, or significant illness, may require temporary dosage adjustments to cope with increased stress on your body.

Important Considerations:

- Salt intake: People with adrenal insufficiency often need to increase their salt intake to maintain adequate sodium levels. Your doctor can provide specific guidelines on how much salt you should consume.
- Potassium levels: It's important to monitor your potassium levels, as mineralocorticoid replacement therapy can sometimes lead to low potassium levels (hypokalemia). Your doctor may need to adjust your dosage or prescribe potassium supplements if necessary.
- Blood pressure monitoring: Regular blood pressure monitoring is crucial, as mineralocorticoid therapy can sometimes cause high blood pressure. Your doctor may need to adjust your dosage or prescribe

additional medications to manage your blood pressure.

By understanding the types of mineralocorticoids, appropriate dosages, monitoring strategies, and potential adjustments, you can work closely with your doctor to optimize your mineralocorticoid replacement therapy and manage your adrenal insufficiency effectively.

Adrenal Androgen Replacement Therapy

Adrenal androgen replacement therapy is a less common aspect of managing adrenal insufficiency, but it can be important for certain individuals, particularly women, who may experience symptoms related to low androgen levels. Androgens are hormones that play a role in various bodily functions, including sexual development and libido.

Types of Androgens:

The type of androgen used for replacement therapy depends on the specific needs of the individual. Some common options include:

- DHEA (dehydroepiandrosterone): This is a precursor hormone that the body can convert into other androgens and estrogens.
- Testosterone: This is the primary male sex hormone, but it can also be used in women to treat low androgen levels.

Dosages:

The dosage of androgen replacement therapy is highly individualized and determined by your doctor based on your specific needs and response to treatment. Factors such as age, sex, symptoms, and underlying health conditions will influence the dosage.

Monitoring:

Regular monitoring is essential to ensure that your androgen replacement therapy is working effectively and safely. This typically involves:

- Blood tests: Blood tests can measure your hormone levels, including androgens, estrogens, and other relevant hormones.

- Physical exams: Your doctor will perform regular physical exams to assess your overall health, including any changes in sexual function, mood, or energy levels.

Adjustments:

Your androgen replacement therapy may require adjustments over time due to various factors:

- Changes in your health: As your body changes or you develop other health conditions, your hormone needs may change.
- Medication interactions: Some medications can interact with androgens, affecting their absorption or metabolism. Your doctor may need to adjust your dosage or consider alternative medications.
- Lifestyle changes: Major lifestyle changes, such as pregnancy, surgery, or significant illness, may require temporary dosage adjustments.

Important Considerations:

- Potential side effects: Androgen therapy can have potential side effects, particularly in women, such as acne, hair growth, and changes in mood. It's important to discuss these risks with your doctor and monitor for any adverse effects.
- Regular monitoring: Regular monitoring of your hormone levels and overall health is crucial to ensure that your therapy is safe and effective.
- Individualized treatment: Androgen replacement therapy is a highly individualized treatment, and your doctor will work with you to determine the best approach for your specific needs.

Surgery and Radiation Therapy

While drug therapy is the primary treatment for adrenal insufficiency, in certain specific cases, surgery or radiation therapy may be considered.

Surgery:

Indications:

- Adrenal tumors: If you have a benign or malignant tumor in one of your adrenal glands, surgery may be necessary to remove the tumor and potentially restore normal adrenal function.
- Adrenal hyperplasia: In some cases of congenital adrenal hyperplasia, surgery may be considered to remove excess adrenal tissue.

Techniques:

- Adrenalectomy: This is a surgical procedure to remove one or both adrenal glands. It's typically performed laparoscopically, a minimally invasive technique that involves small incisions and a camera to guide the surgeon.

Complications:

- Adrenal insufficiency: After surgery to remove one or both adrenal glands, you will need lifelong hormone replacement therapy to manage adrenal insufficiency.

- Infection: As with any surgery, there is a risk of infection at the surgical site.
- Bleeding: Excessive bleeding can occur during or after surgery.
- Injury to nearby organs: There is a small risk of injury to nearby organs, such as the kidneys or liver, during surgery.

Radiation Therapy:

Indications:

- Inoperable adrenal tumors: If a tumor is inoperable, radiation therapy may be used to shrink the tumor and control its growth.
- Adrenal cancer that has spread: Radiation therapy may be used to relieve symptoms and slow the progression of cancer that has spread to other parts of the body.

Techniques:

- External beam radiation therapy: This involves directing high-energy radiation beams at the adrenal gland tumor from a machine outside the body.

Complications:

- Fatigue: Radiation therapy can cause fatigue and weakness.
- Skin irritation: The skin in the treatment area may become irritated and red.
- Digestive issues: Radiation therapy can affect the digestive system, leading to nausea, vomiting, and diarrhea.
- Increased risk of other cancers: Long-term exposure to radiation can increase the risk of developing other types of cancer.

It's important to note that surgery and radiation therapy are not typically first-line treatments for adrenal insufficiency. They are usually considered only in specific cases and after careful evaluation by a specialist. If you are considering surgery or radiation therapy, it's crucial to discuss the potential benefits and risks with your doctor.

Lifestyle Modifications

In addition to medical treatment, lifestyle modifications can play a significant role in managing adrenal insufficiency. By making certain adjustments to your diet, exercise routine, stress management techniques, and sleep habits, you can improve your overall well-being and help manage the symptoms of your condition.

Diet

- Balanced diet: A balanced diet rich in fruits, vegetables, whole grains, and lean protein can provide essential nutrients to support your body's functions.
- Adequate salt intake: People with adrenal insufficiency may need to increase their salt intake to maintain healthy sodium levels. Consult your doctor for specific recommendations.
- Hydration: Staying hydrated is important for overall health. Drink plenty of water throughout the day.

- Limit caffeine and alcohol: Excessive caffeine and alcohol consumption can disrupt sleep and affect hormone levels.
- Avoid excessive sugar: High sugar intake can lead to blood sugar fluctuations and may exacerbate symptoms of adrenal insufficiency.

Exercise

- Regular physical activity: Regular exercise can help improve energy levels, reduce stress, and boost mood. However, it's important to listen to your body and avoid overexertion.
- Low-impact exercises: Low-impact exercises like walking, swimming, and yoga are generally well-tolerated and can be beneficial.
- Avoid intense exercise during stress: Intense exercise during periods of stress can further strain your adrenal glands.
- Listen to your body: If you feel fatigued or unwell, take a break and rest.

Stress Management

- Stress reduction techniques: Practice stress-reduction techniques like meditation, deep breathing, or yoga to help manage stress and anxiety.
- Time management: Effective time management can help reduce stress and improve overall well-being.
- Prioritize tasks: Prioritize tasks and avoid overcommitting yourself.
- Seek support: Talk to friends, family, or a therapist about your feelings and challenges.

Sleep Hygiene

- Consistent sleep schedule: Try to go to bed and wake up at the same time each day, even on weekends.
- Create a relaxing bedtime routine: Establish a relaxing bedtime routine to signal to your body that it's time to wind down.
- Optimize your sleep environment: Make sure your bedroom is dark, quiet, and cool.

- Limit screen time before bed: The blue light emitted by electronic devices can interfere with sleep.
- Avoid stimulants before bed: Avoid caffeine and alcohol, especially in the evening.

By incorporating these lifestyle modifications into your daily routine, you can improve your overall well-being and manage the symptoms of adrenal insufficiency more effectively. Remember to consult with your doctor before making significant changes to your diet or exercise routine.

Emergency Management

Adrenal crisis is a life-threatening condition that can occur in people with adrenal insufficiency when their cortisol levels drop dangerously low. Prompt recognition and treatment are crucial to prevent serious complications.

Adrenal Crisis Treatment

Immediate Treatment:

- Hydrocortisone Injection: This is the primary treatment for adrenal crisis. It involves a rapid intravenous or intramuscular injection of hydrocortisone, a synthetic form of cortisol.
- Fluid Replacement: Intravenous fluids, such as saline, are administered to replace fluids lost due to dehydration.
- Electrolyte Correction: Blood tests are performed to check electrolyte levels, and intravenous fluids containing electrolytes, such as sodium and potassium, may be given to correct imbalances.

Ongoing Management:

- Hospitalization: Most people with adrenal crisis require hospitalization for close monitoring and treatment.
- Continuous Monitoring: Blood pressure, heart rate, and blood sugar levels are monitored closely.
- Additional Medications: Depending on the severity of the crisis and individual needs, additional medications may be required, such

as medications to increase blood pressure or regulate heart rhythm.

Adrenal Crisis Prevention

Adherence to Treatment:

- Regular Medication: It's crucial to take your prescribed glucocorticoid and mineralocorticoid medications as directed by your doctor.
- Stress Dosing: During periods of significant stress, such as illness, surgery, or emotional distress, you may need to increase your glucocorticoid dosage temporarily. Consult your doctor for specific guidance.
- Emergency Kit: Carry an emergency kit containing injectable hydrocortisone and instructions on how to administer it in case of a crisis.

Recognizing Symptoms:

- Early Signs: Be aware of the early signs of an adrenal crisis, such as severe fatigue, weakness, nausea, vomiting, abdominal pain, low blood pressure, and confusion.

- Seek Immediate Medical Attention: If you experience these symptoms, seek immediate medical attention.

Education and Preparedness:

- Inform Loved Ones: Educate your family and friends about adrenal insufficiency and how to recognize the signs of an adrenal crisis.
- Wear a Medical Alert Bracelet: Consider wearing a medical alert bracelet or necklace to inform medical personnel about your condition in case of an emergency.

By understanding the signs and symptoms of adrenal crisis, adhering to your treatment plan, and being prepared for emergencies, you can significantly reduce your risk of experiencing a life-threatening crisis.

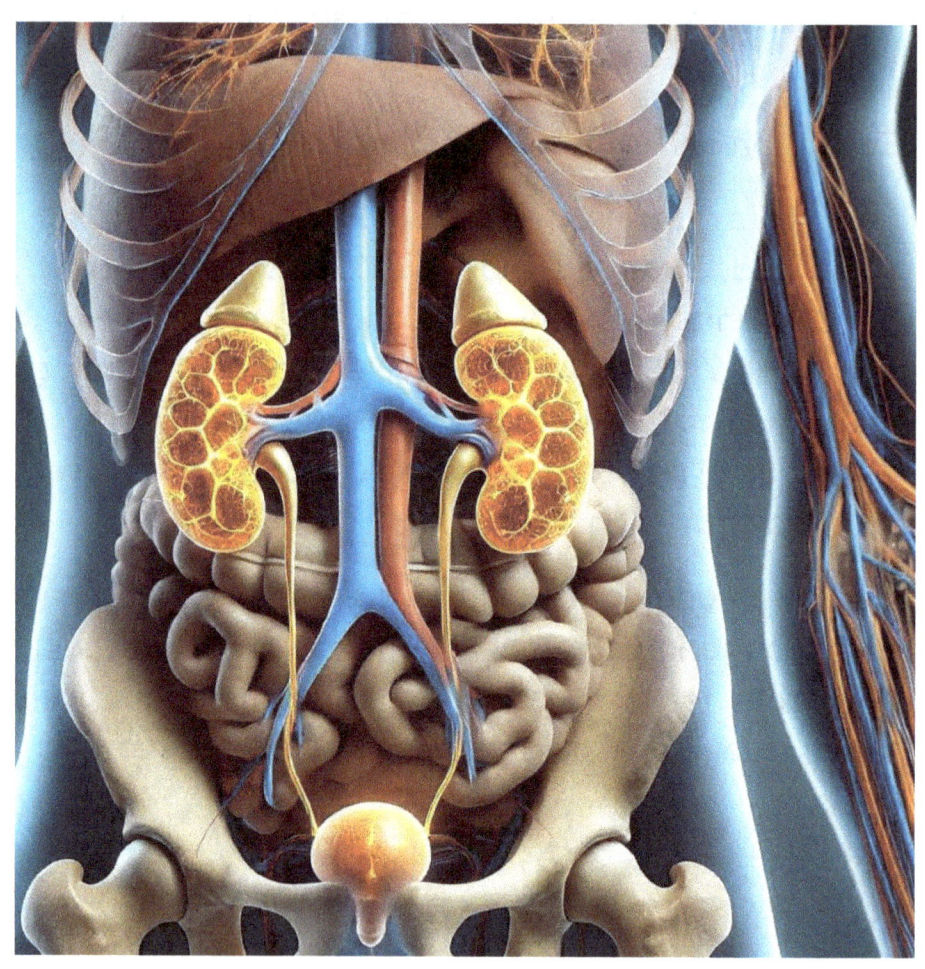

Part 7: Special Considerations

Pediatric Adrenal Insufficiency

In children, AI can have significant health implications, affecting growth, development, and overall well-being. This comprehensive guide will delve into the diagnosis, treatment, management, and growth considerations of pediatric adrenal insufficiency.

Diagnosis of Pediatric Adrenal Insufficiency

Diagnosing adrenal insufficiency in children requires a careful evaluation of symptoms and laboratory tests. Common symptoms include:

- Fatigue and weakness
- Abdominal pain
- Nausea and vomiting
- Weight loss
- Dehydration
- Low blood pressure
- Salt craving
- Skin darkening (hyperpigmentation)

Laboratory tests to confirm the diagnosis include:

- Cosyntropin Stimulation Test: This test measures the body's response to synthetic ACTH (adrenocorticotropic hormone). In adrenal insufficiency, cortisol levels fail to rise appropriately after the injection of cosyntropin.
- ACTH Level: This test measures the level of ACTH in the blood. In primary adrenal insufficiency, ACTH levels are usually elevated.
- Electrolyte Levels: This test measures the levels of sodium, potassium, and other electrolytes in the blood. Abnormalities in electrolyte levels can be seen in adrenal insufficiency.

Treatment of Pediatric Adrenal Insufficiency

The primary treatment for adrenal insufficiency is hormone replacement therapy, which involves taking medications to replace the missing hormones. The most common medications used are:

- Hydrocortisone: This medication replaces cortisol, the primary hormone produced by the adrenal glands. It is typically taken in divided doses throughout the day.

- Fludrocortisone: This medication replaces aldosterone, a hormone that helps regulate blood pressure and fluid balance. It is usually taken once daily.

Management of Pediatric Adrenal Insufficiency

Managing adrenal insufficiency in children requires a multidisciplinary approach involving endocrinologists, pediatricians, and other healthcare professionals. Key management strategies include:

- Regular Monitoring: Children with adrenal insufficiency require regular monitoring of their hormone levels, blood pressure, and electrolyte levels.
- Stress Dosing: During times of stress, such as illness, surgery, or injury, children with adrenal insufficiency may need additional doses of hydrocortisone to prevent adrenal crisis.
- Education and Support: Education and support for children and their families are

essential to ensure proper management of the condition. This includes teaching children and their families how to recognize and respond to symptoms of adrenal crisis, administer medications correctly, and adjust their medication doses during times of stress.

- Medical Alert Bracelets: Children with adrenal insufficiency should wear medical alert bracelets to inform healthcare providers about their condition in case of an emergency.

Growth Considerations in Pediatric Adrenal Insufficiency

Adrenal insufficiency can affect growth and development in children. Cortisol plays a crucial role in growth hormone production, and inadequate cortisol levels can lead to growth delays. Early diagnosis and treatment of adrenal insufficiency are essential to optimize growth and development.

Children with adrenal insufficiency may require additional growth hormone therapy to achieve optimal growth. Regular monitoring of growth parameters, including height, weight, and bone age, is important to assess the child's growth trajectory and adjust treatment as needed.

Adrenal Insufficiency in Pregnancy

Adrenal insufficiency (AI), can pose significant risks during pregnancy. Understanding these risks, implementing appropriate monitoring strategies, and providing effective management are crucial for ensuring the well-being of both the mother and the fetus.

Risks of Adrenal Insufficiency in Pregnancy

- Adrenal Crisis: This life-threatening condition can occur if the body doesn't produce enough cortisol, a hormone essential for managing stress. Pregnancy is a period of physiological stress, increasing the risk of adrenal crisis in women with AI.
- Gestational Hypertension: High blood pressure during pregnancy is more common in women with AI, potentially leading to complications like preeclampsia.

- Preterm Labor: AI can increase the risk of early labor and delivery.
- Intrauterine Growth Restriction (IUGR): This condition, where the fetus doesn't grow at the expected rate, can occur in pregnancies complicated by AI.
- Fetal Adrenal Insufficiency: In rare cases, AI can be inherited, and the fetus may also be affected, leading to complications such as fetal distress and stillbirth.

Monitoring Adrenal Insufficiency During Pregnancy

Close monitoring is essential to manage AI during pregnancy. This typically involves:

- Regular Check-ups: Frequent visits to the doctor to assess the mother's health and the baby's growth.
- Blood Tests: Monitoring hormone levels, electrolyte levels, and kidney function.
- Ultrasound Scans: To assess fetal growth and development.

- Non-Stress Tests (NSTs): To monitor the baby's heart rate and response to movement.
- Biophysical Profiles (BPPs): A comprehensive assessment of the fetus's well-being, including heart rate, breathing movements, fetal movement, fetal tone, and amniotic fluid volume.

Management of Adrenal Insufficiency in Pregnancy

Effective management of AI during pregnancy is crucial to minimize risks and optimize outcomes. Strategies include:

- Hormone Replacement Therapy: Adjusting medication dosages to ensure adequate hormone levels throughout pregnancy. This may involve increasing the dose of hydrocortisone, particularly during periods of stress or illness.
- Dietary Modifications: A well-balanced diet, rich in sodium, is essential to maintain electrolyte balance.

- Stress Management: Strategies to reduce stress, such as relaxation techniques and adequate sleep, can help prevent adrenal crises.
- Close Monitoring: Regular monitoring of the mother's health and fetal well-being is essential.
- Early Delivery: In some cases, early delivery may be considered if the pregnancy is complicated by severe AI or fetal distress.

Fetal Implications of Adrenal Insufficiency in Pregnancy

As mentioned earlier, fetal adrenal insufficiency is a rare but serious complication. If the fetus is affected, it may experience:

- Intrauterine Growth Restriction (IUGR): The fetus may not grow at the expected rate.
- Fetal Distress: Reduced oxygen supply to the fetus.
- Stillbirth: In severe cases, fetal death may occur.

Early diagnosis and close monitoring of the fetus are essential to identify potential complications and intervene promptly. In some cases, fetal surgery may be considered to treat congenital adrenal hyperplasia, a condition that can lead to fetal adrenal insufficiency.

Adrenal insufficiency in pregnancy requires careful management to ensure the well-being of both the mother and the fetus. By understanding the risks, implementing appropriate monitoring strategies, and providing effective treatment, healthcare providers can optimize outcomes for women with AI and their babies. Regular check-ups, hormone replacement therapy, dietary modifications, stress management, and close monitoring are essential components of managing AI during pregnancy.

Adrenal Insufficiency in Elderly

Adrenal insufficiency (AI) in the elderly population presents unique challenges due to age-related physiological changes, the presence of comorbidities, and the complexity of polypharmacy. Understanding these factors is crucial for accurate diagnosis, appropriate management, and improved outcomes.

Age-Related Considerations

As individuals age, the adrenal glands undergo physiological changes that can influence the presentation and course of AI. These changes include:

- Decreased Adrenal Reserve: The ability of the adrenal glands to respond to stress may diminish with age. This reduced reserve can make older adults more susceptible to adrenal crisis, even in response to minor stressors.
- Altered Hormone Regulation: Age-related changes in the hypothalamic-pituitary-adrenal (HPA) axis can affect the production and regulation of cortisol. This can lead to subtle or atypical presentations of AI in older adults.
- Increased Sensitivity to Cortisol: Elderly individuals may be more sensitive to the

effects of cortisol, making them more prone to side effects of hormone replacement therapy, such as osteoporosis and diabetes.

Comorbidities

The presence of comorbidities, common in the elderly population, can complicate the diagnosis and management of AI. Some common comorbidities that can interact with AI include:

- Cardiovascular Disease: AI can contribute to cardiovascular complications, such as heart failure and arrhythmias.
- Diabetes Mellitus: Both conditions can share similar symptoms, making diagnosis challenging. Additionally, diabetes can affect the body's response to stress and influence cortisol levels.
- Chronic Kidney Disease: Kidney dysfunction can impair the production and metabolism of hormones, including cortisol.
- Autoimmune Diseases: Autoimmune diseases, such as rheumatoid arthritis and systemic lupus erythematosus, are more prevalent in older adults and can increase the risk of AI.

Polypharmacy

Polypharmacy, the use of multiple medications, is common in the elderly population and can significantly impact the management of AI. Several medications can interact with cortisol metabolism or adrenal function, potentially exacerbating AI or masking its symptoms.

- Corticosteroids: Long-term use of corticosteroids can suppress the HPA axis, leading to secondary adrenal insufficiency.
- Nonsteroidal Anti-Inflammatory Drugs (NSAIDs): NSAIDs can interfere with renal function and electrolyte balance, which can impact the management of AI.
- Diuretics: Diuretics can lead to electrolyte imbalances, particularly hypokalemia, which can worsen AI.

Adrenal insufficiency in the elderly population presents unique challenges due to age-related changes, comorbidities, and polypharmacy. Recognizing the atypical presentations, considering the impact of comorbidities, and carefully managing medication interactions are crucial for accurate diagnosis and effective management of AI in older adults. By addressing these factors, healthcare providers can improve the quality of life and overall health of elderly individuals with AI.

Psychological and Emotional Aspects

Adrenal insufficiency (AI) is not only a physical condition but can also have a significant impact on a person's emotional well-being. Understanding the psychological aspects of AI can help individuals cope with the challenges and improve their overall quality of life.

The Psychological Impact of AI

Living with a chronic condition like AI can be emotionally taxing. Some common psychological challenges faced by individuals with AI include:

- Anxiety and Stress: The fear of adrenal crisis, a life-threatening condition that can occur if cortisol levels drop too low, can cause significant anxiety and stress.

- Fatigue and Low Energy: The constant fatigue associated with AI can impact mood, motivation, and overall quality of life.
- Depression: Chronic illness can contribute to feelings of sadness, hopelessness, and worthlessness.
- Social Isolation: The physical limitations and emotional challenges of AI can lead to social withdrawal and isolation.

Coping Mechanisms

To manage the psychological impact of AI, individuals can employ various coping mechanisms:

- Education and Self-Management: Learning about AI, understanding its symptoms, and developing a personalized management plan can empower individuals to take control of their condition.
- Stress Management Techniques: Practices like mindfulness meditation, yoga, and deep breathing can help reduce stress and anxiety.

- Regular Exercise: Physical activity can improve mood, energy levels, and overall well-being.
- Healthy Diet: A balanced diet can provide the necessary nutrients to support physical and mental health.
- Adequate Sleep: Prioritizing sleep can help manage fatigue and improve mood.
- Seeking Professional Help: Therapy can provide a safe space to discuss feelings, develop coping strategies, and address mental health concerns.

Support Groups

Connecting with others who understand the challenges of living with AI can be incredibly beneficial. Support groups provide a supportive environment where individuals can share experiences, offer advice, and reduce feelings of isolation.

- Online Support Groups: Online forums and social media groups allow individuals to connect with others from around the world.

- Local Support Groups: In-person support groups offer opportunities for face-to-face interaction and building relationships with others in the community.

Mental Health

It's important to prioritize mental health when living with AI. If you're struggling with anxiety, depression, or other mental health concerns, don't hesitate to seek professional help. A mental health professional can provide therapy, medication, or other interventions to help you manage your symptoms and improve your overall well-being.

By understanding the psychological impact of AI, employing effective coping mechanisms, seeking support from others, and prioritizing mental health, individuals with AI can improve their quality of life and live fulfilling lives. Remember, you're not alone, and help is available.

Traveling and Vaccination Considerations

Traveling with adrenal insufficiency (AI) requires careful planning and preparation to ensure a safe and enjoyable experience. By taking necessary precautions, following recommendations, and being prepared for emergencies, individuals with AI can confidently explore the world.

Precautions

- Consult Your Doctor: Before any trip, consult with your endocrinologist to discuss your specific needs and any necessary adjustments to your medication regimen.
- Inform Your Travel Companions: Make sure your travel companions are aware of your condition and are prepared to assist you in case of an emergency.
- Pack Essential Medications: Ensure you have an adequate supply of all your medications, including hydrocortisone and fludrocortisone. Pack them in your carry-on luggage to avoid potential loss or damage.

- Carry a Medical Alert Bracelet or Card: This will alert healthcare professionals to your condition in case of an emergency.
- Consider Travel Insurance: Having comprehensive travel insurance can provide peace of mind and cover unexpected medical expenses.

Recommendations

- Choose Your Destination Wisely: Consider factors such as climate, altitude, and access to medical care when planning your trip. Avoid destinations with extreme climates or limited healthcare facilities.
- Pack a Medical Kit: Include essential items like glucose tablets, electrolyte solutions, syringes, and alcohol swabs.
- Stay Hydrated: Dehydration can exacerbate the symptoms of AI, so it's important to drink plenty of fluids, especially in hot climates.
- Eat Regularly: Maintain regular meal times to avoid hypoglycemia, which can worsen symptoms.

- Monitor Your Blood Sugar: If you have diabetes, monitor your blood sugar levels regularly and adjust your insulin or oral medication as needed.
- Be Mindful of Time Zone Changes: Time zone changes can disrupt your circadian rhythm and affect hormone levels. Adjust your medication schedule accordingly.
- Avoid Unnecessary Stress: Stress can trigger adrenal crises, so try to relax and manage stress effectively.

Emergency Preparedness

- Carry an Emergency Kit: This kit should include extra doses of your medications, a glucose meter, glucose tablets, insulin (if applicable), and a list of your medications and dosages.
- Know the Signs of Adrenal Crisis: Be aware of the symptoms of adrenal crisis, such as severe fatigue, nausea, vomiting, abdominal pain, low blood pressure, and confusion.

- Have a Plan for Emergencies: Know how to contact emergency services in your destination country and have a list of local hospitals and clinics.
- Consider a Travel Buddy: Having a travel companion can provide support and assistance, especially in unfamiliar situations.

By following these precautions, recommendations, and emergency preparedness tips, individuals with AI can travel safely and confidently. Remember to consult with your healthcare provider to create a personalized travel plan that meets your specific needs.

Part 8: Complications and Prognosis

Short Term Complications

Adrenal insufficiency can lead to several short-term complications. These can be life-threatening and require immediate medical attention. Here's a closer look at some of the most common ones:

Adrenal Crisis

An adrenal crisis, also known as Addisonian crisis, is a medical emergency that occurs when your body experiences severe stress, such as illness, injury, or surgery. During these times, your body needs more cortisol, a hormone produced by your adrenal glands. However, with adrenal insufficiency, your body can't produce enough cortisol to meet this increased demand. This can lead to a rapid decline in your health and potentially life-threatening consequences.

Symptoms of an adrenal crisis include:

- Severe fatigue and weakness
- Severe abdominal, back, or leg pain
- Severe vomiting and diarrhea
- Low blood pressure
- Rapid, weak pulse
- Loss of consciousness

If you experience any of these symptoms, seek immediate medical attention.

Electrolyte Imbalance

Your adrenal glands play a crucial role in regulating your body's electrolyte levels, including sodium, potassium, and chloride. When your adrenal glands aren't functioning properly, it can lead to imbalances in these electrolytes.

- Hyponatremia: This occurs when your sodium levels are too low. Symptoms can include fatigue, confusion, muscle weakness, and seizures.
- Hyperkalemia: This occurs when your potassium levels are too high. Symptoms can

include muscle weakness, irregular heartbeat, and in severe cases, cardiac arrest.

Hypoglycemia

The adrenal glands help regulate blood sugar levels by releasing cortisol in response to stress. When your adrenal glands are underactive, your body may not produce enough cortisol to raise your blood sugar levels, leading to hypoglycemia (low blood sugar).

Symptoms of hypoglycemia include:

- Shakiness
- Sweating
- Anxiety
- Hunger
- Confusion
- Difficulty concentrating
- Blurred vision
- Seizures
- Loss of consciousness

Hypotension

Your adrenal glands produce aldosterone, a hormone that helps regulate blood pressure. When your adrenal glands are underactive, your body may not produce enough aldosterone, leading to hypotension (low blood pressure).

Symptoms of hypotension include:

- Dizziness
- Lightheadedness
- Fatigue
- Blurred vision
- Fainting

Long Term Complications

While adrenal insufficiency can lead to immediate and life-threatening complications, it can also have long-term consequences if left untreated. Here's a look at some of the potential long-term complications:

Osteoporosis

Adrenal insufficiency can lead to reduced bone mineral density, increasing the risk of osteoporosis. Cortisol, a hormone produced by the adrenal glands, plays a crucial role in maintaining bone health. When cortisol levels are low, it can lead to bone loss and increased risk of fractures.

Hypertension

While adrenal insufficiency is often associated with low blood pressure, it can also lead to high blood pressure (hypertension) in some individuals. This can occur due to various factors, including electrolyte imbalances and the body's compensatory mechanisms to maintain blood pressure.

Diabetes

Adrenal insufficiency can increase the risk of developing type 2 diabetes. Cortisol plays a role in regulating blood sugar levels, and when cortisol levels are low, it can lead to insulin resistance and impaired glucose tolerance.

Cardiovascular Diseases

Adrenal insufficiency can increase the risk of cardiovascular diseases, such as heart attack and stroke. This is due to a combination of factors, including electrolyte imbalances, high blood pressure, and increased risk of blood clots.

Other potential long-term complications of adrenal insufficiency include:

- Fatigue and weakness: Persistent fatigue and weakness can significantly impact your quality of life.
- Mental health issues: Adrenal insufficiency can contribute to mood disorders, such as depression and anxiety.
- Weight gain: Some individuals with adrenal insufficiency may experience weight gain, particularly in the abdominal area.
- Skin problems: Skin problems, such as dry skin, hyperpigmentation, and poor wound healing, can occur.
- Muscle weakness: Muscle weakness can lead to difficulty with daily activities and increased risk of falls.

It's important to note that the risk of these long-term complications can be significantly reduced with proper treatment and management of adrenal insufficiency.

Prognosis and Quality of Life

With proper management and adherence to treatment, individuals with adrenal insufficiency can live long and fulfilling lives. The prognosis for individuals with adrenal insufficiency has significantly improved over the years, thanks to advancements in diagnosis and treatment.

Prognosis with Proper Management

- Life Expectancy: With appropriate treatment, most individuals with adrenal insufficiency can expect a normal life expectancy.
- Reduced Risk of Complications: Consistent medication adherence and regular monitoring can significantly reduce the risk of acute adrenal crises and other complications.
- Improved Quality of Life: Effective treatment can help alleviate symptoms such as fatigue, weakness, and mood disturbances, leading to a better quality of life.

Factors Affecting Prognosis

Several factors can influence the prognosis of individuals with adrenal insufficiency:

- Adherence to Treatment: Consistent medication adherence is crucial for maintaining hormone levels and preventing complications.
- Regular Monitoring: Regular monitoring of hormone levels, electrolyte levels, and blood pressure helps ensure optimal treatment and early detection of potential problems.
- Prompt Treatment of Acute Crises: Timely and appropriate treatment of adrenal crises is essential to prevent life-threatening complications.
- Management of Underlying Conditions: If adrenal insufficiency is secondary to another condition, managing the underlying condition is important for overall health.

Quality of Life with Adrenal Insufficiency

While adrenal insufficiency can present challenges, many individuals with the condition can maintain a good quality of life with proper management. Here are some tips for improving quality of life:

- Adherence to Treatment: Consistent medication adherence is essential for managing symptoms and preventing complications.
- Stress Management: Learning effective stress management techniques can help minimize the impact of stress on the body and reduce the risk of adrenal crises.
- Healthy Lifestyle: A healthy diet, regular exercise, and adequate sleep can contribute to overall well-being.
- Medical Alert: Wearing a medical alert bracelet or necklace can alert healthcare providers to your condition in case of an emergency.
- Education and Support: Staying informed about your condition and seeking support from healthcare providers and support groups can help you manage your condition effectively.

Future Directions

While significant progress has been made in the management of adrenal insufficiency, ongoing research continues to explore new avenues for improving treatment and quality of life for affected individuals. Here are some promising future directions:

Emerging Therapies

1. Novel Drug Development: Researchers are actively investigating new medications that can more effectively mimic the actions of cortisol and aldosterone. These drugs may offer improved efficacy and fewer side effects compared to current treatments.
2. Targeted Therapies: By identifying specific molecular targets involved in adrenal insufficiency, researchers aim to develop targeted therapies that can address the underlying causes of the condition.
3. Gene Therapy: Gene therapy holds the potential to correct genetic defects that lead

to adrenal insufficiency. While still in its early stages, this approach offers hope for a long-term cure for certain forms of the disease.

Potential Breakthroughs

1. Personalized Medicine: Advances in genomics and personalized medicine may allow for tailored treatment plans based on an individual's genetic makeup and specific needs.
2. Improved Monitoring Devices: The development of advanced monitoring devices, such as continuous glucose monitors and wearable sensors, can help individuals with adrenal insufficiency track their hormone levels and adjust their treatment accordingly.
3. Artificial Pancreas-like Devices: Inspired by artificial pancreas technology used for diabetes management, researchers are exploring the possibility of developing devices that can automatically deliver hormones as needed, reducing the burden of frequent injections.

Ongoing Research Areas

1. Understanding the Pathophysiology of Adrenal Insufficiency: Continued research into the underlying mechanisms of adrenal insufficiency can lead to new insights into disease pathogenesis and identify novel therapeutic targets.
2. Identifying Early Biomarkers: Early identification of individuals at risk for adrenal insufficiency can facilitate timely intervention and prevent complications.
3. Improving Patient Education and Support: Enhancing patient education and support programs can empower individuals with adrenal insufficiency to manage their condition effectively and improve their quality of life.

As research progresses, we can anticipate exciting advancements in the field of adrenal insufficiency. These developments hold the promise of improving the lives of individuals affected by this condition and ultimately leading to a cure.

Part 9: Appendices

Glossary of Terms

Basic Terms

- Adrenal Glands: Two small glands located on top of each kidney.
- Adrenal Cortex: The outer layer of the adrenal gland, responsible for producing cortisol, aldosterone, and sex hormones.
- Adrenal Medulla: The inner layer of the adrenal gland, responsible for producing adrenaline (epinephrine) and noradrenaline (norepinephrine).
- Hormone: A chemical messenger produced by glands and released into the bloodstream to regulate various bodily functions.
- Endocrine System: A system of glands that secrete hormones directly into the bloodstream.

Specific Terms Related to Adrenal Insufficiency

- Adrenal Insufficiency (AI): A condition where the adrenal glands don't produce enough cortisol and, sometimes, aldosterone.
- Primary Adrenal Insufficiency (Addison's Disease): A condition where the adrenal glands themselves are damaged or dysfunctional.
- Secondary Adrenal Insufficiency: A condition where the pituitary gland doesn't produce enough adrenocorticotropic hormone (ACTH), leading to decreased cortisol production.
- Tertiary Adrenal Insufficiency: A condition where the hypothalamus doesn't produce enough corticotropin-releasing hormone (CRH), affecting the pituitary gland and leading to decreased cortisol production.
- Adrenocorticotropic Hormone (ACTH): A hormone produced by the pituitary gland that stimulates the adrenal cortex to produce cortisol.
- Cortisol: A hormone produced by the adrenal cortex that helps regulate stress, blood sugar levels, blood pressure, and immune function.

- Aldosterone: A hormone produced by the adrenal cortex that helps regulate blood pressure and fluid balance.
- Hydrocortisone: A synthetic form of cortisol used as medication to treat adrenal insufficiency.
- Fludrocortisone: A synthetic form of aldosterone used as medication to treat adrenal insufficiency, particularly in cases of low blood pressure.

Symptoms and Complications

- Fatigue: Persistent tiredness and weakness.
- Muscle Weakness: Difficulty with physical activity.
- Weight Loss: Unintentional weight loss, often accompanied by decreased appetite.
- Low Blood Pressure (Hypotension): Dizziness, lightheadedness, or fainting.
- Low Blood Sugar (Hypoglycemia): Symptoms like sweating, shakiness, and confusion.
- Salt Cravings: A desire for salty foods due to low sodium levels.

- Nausea and Vomiting: Digestive disturbances.
- Skin Hyperpigmentation: Darkening of the skin, particularly in areas of sun exposure.
- Adrenal Crisis: A life-threatening condition characterized by severe symptoms of adrenal insufficiency, including shock, rapid heart rate, and low blood pressure.

Diagnosis and Treatment

- Blood Tests: Measuring cortisol levels and ACTH levels.
- Cosyntropin Stimulation Test: A test to assess the adrenal gland's response to ACTH.
- Hormone Replacement Therapy (HRT): Treatment with hydrocortisone and, in some cases, fludrocortisone.
- Stress Dose Cortisol: Additional doses of cortisol during periods of stress or illness.
- Medical Alert Bracelet: A bracelet indicating the condition and necessary emergency treatment.

Autoimmune Diseases:

- Autoimmune Diseases: Conditions where the body's immune system mistakenly attacks its own tissues.
- Autoimmune Adrenalitis: An autoimmune disease that targets the adrenal glands, leading to primary adrenal insufficiency.

Medications and Treatments:

- Steroid Medications: Synthetic hormones like hydrocortisone and prednisone used to replace missing cortisol.
- Mineralocorticoid Medications: Medications like fludrocortisone used to replace missing aldosterone.
- Stress Dosing: Increasing medication dosage during periods of physical or emotional stress.
- Adrenal Crisis Kit: A kit containing emergency medications to treat an adrenal crisis.

Lifestyle and Management:

- Medical Alert Bracelet: A bracelet indicating the condition and necessary emergency treatment.

- Diet: A balanced diet with adequate sodium intake to maintain blood pressure.
- Hydration: Staying hydrated to prevent dehydration, especially during illness or increased stress.
- Regular Medical Check-ups: Monitoring hormone levels and overall health.
- Stress Management: Techniques like meditation, yoga, or deep breathing to manage stress.

Research and Future Directions:

- Genetic Factors: Investigating genetic predispositions to adrenal insufficiency.
- Novel Therapies: Exploring new treatments, including potential gene therapies.
- Improved Patient Education and Support: Enhancing awareness and providing resources for patients and caregivers.

Resources and Support Groups

National Organizations

- National Adrenal Diseases Foundation (NADF): A non-profit organization dedicated to providing information, education, and support to patients diagnosed with adrenal diseases. They offer support groups, educational materials, and a helpline.
    - Website: https://www.nadf.us/
- Adrenal Insufficiency United: This organization is committed to enhancing the lives and health of individuals with adrenal insufficiency through awareness, support, and advocacy.
    - Website: https://aiunited.org/

Online Communities and Support Groups

- Social Media: Join online groups on platforms like Facebook and Reddit to connect with others living with adrenal insufficiency. Search for groups using keywords like "Addison's Disease," "Adrenal Insufficiency," or "Endocrine Disorders."
- Online Forums: Participate in online forums and message boards where you can share

experiences, ask questions, and receive support from others.

- Patient Advocacy Groups: Consider joining patient advocacy groups that focus on rare diseases or endocrine disorders. These groups often have online communities and resources.

Healthcare Professionals

- Endocrinologist: A specialist in hormone disorders. They can provide diagnosis, treatment, and ongoing management of adrenal insufficiency.
- Primary Care Physician: Your primary care physician can work with an endocrinologist to manage your condition.
- Nurse Practitioner: Nurse practitioners can provide education, support, and manage certain aspects of your care.

Additional Resources

- Books and Publications: Explore books and articles on adrenal insufficiency to gain knowledge and support.

- Mobile Apps: Use mobile apps to track symptoms, medication, and blood sugar levels.
- Local Support Groups: Check with your local hospital or community center for in-person support groups.
- Online Support Groups: Participate in online support groups to connect with others living with adrenal insufficiency.

Hotlines and Help Lines

- National Adrenal Diseases Foundation (NADF) Helpline: While specific hotline numbers may change, you can contact the NADF for information and support. Check their website or social media for the most up-to-date contact information.

Important Considerations

- Advocate for Yourself: Don't hesitate to ask questions and seek clarification from your healthcare provider.
- Stay Informed: Keep up-to-date on the latest research and treatment options.

- Take Care of Yourself: Prioritize self-care, including stress management, healthy eating, and adequate sleep.
- Connect with Others: Building relationships with other individuals with adrenal insufficiency can provide valuable support and understanding.

Remember: The landscape of online resources and support groups is constantly evolving. It's always a good idea to check for the latest information and updates.

Medication Lists

Medications commonly used in the management of adrenal insufficiency include:

1. Glucocorticoids:

- Hydrocortisone: The most commonly prescribed medication to replace cortisol, the primary hormone produced by the adrenal glands. It is typically taken in divided doses throughout the day to mimic the body's natural cortisol production.

- Prednisone: A stronger glucocorticoid that may be used in certain situations, such as during acute stress or illness. It is often prescribed in higher doses for shorter periods.

- Dexamethasone: A very potent glucocorticoid that is used in specific situations, such as adrenal crises or to suppress inflammation. It is generally not used for long-term replacement therapy.

2. Mineralocorticoids:

- Fludrocortisone: This medication replaces aldosterone, another hormone produced by the adrenal glands that helps regulate blood pressure and fluid balance. It is typically taken once daily.

Important Considerations:

- Dosage and Timing: The dosage and timing of these medications are individualized and determined by your doctor based on your specific needs. It is crucial to follow your doctor's instructions carefully.

- Stress Dosing: During periods of physical or emotional stress, such as illness, surgery, or trauma, you may need to increase your medication dosage temporarily. This is known as "stress dosing" and is essential to prevent adrenal crisis.

- Regular Monitoring: Regular monitoring of your hormone levels, blood pressure, and electrolyte levels is important to ensure that your medication dosage is appropriate and effective.

- Side Effects: Like any medication, glucocorticoids and mineralocorticoids can have potential side effects. It is important to discuss these with your doctor and monitor for any adverse effects.

Additional Medications:

In some cases, additional medications may be prescribed to manage specific symptoms or complications associated with adrenal insufficiency. These may include:

- Antibiotics: To treat infections.
- Anti-nausea medications: To manage nausea and vomiting.
- Anti-seizure medications: In rare cases of severe electrolyte imbalances.

It is important to remember that this is not an exhaustive list of medications used in adrenal insufficiency. Your doctor will determine the most appropriate medications and dosage for your individual needs.

Laboratory Test Reference Ranges

Laboratory tests play a crucial role in diagnosing and monitoring adrenal insufficiency. Here are some of the key tests used:

1. Cortisol Level:

- Normal Range: The normal range for cortisol levels can vary depending on the laboratory, but generally, it's between 5-25 mcg/dL in the morning.
- Interpretation:
    - Low cortisol levels, especially in the morning, are indicative of adrenal insufficiency.
    - Elevated cortisol levels can rule out adrenal insufficiency but may suggest other conditions like Cushing's syndrome.
- Critical Values:
    - Very low cortisol levels can be a medical emergency and may require immediate treatment.

2. Adrenocorticotropic Hormone (ACTH) Level:

- Normal Range: The normal range for ACTH levels is 10-60 pg/mL.
- Interpretation:
  - Elevated ACTH levels in the presence of low cortisol levels strongly suggest primary adrenal insufficiency (Addison's disease).
  - Low ACTH levels with low cortisol levels may indicate secondary or tertiary adrenal insufficiency.
- Critical Values:
  - Not typically applicable.

3. Cosyntropin Stimulation Test:

- Procedure: This test involves administering synthetic ACTH (cosyntropin) intravenously and measuring cortisol levels before and after administration.
- Interpretation:
  - A normal response is a significant increase in cortisol levels after cosyntropin administration.

- A blunted response suggests adrenal insufficiency.
- Critical Values:
  - Not typically applicable.

4. Aldosterone Level:

- Normal Range: The normal range for aldosterone levels varies depending on the laboratory and the patient's sodium intake.
- Interpretation:
  - Low aldosterone levels can indicate adrenal insufficiency, particularly in cases of primary adrenal insufficiency.
- Critical Values:
  - Not typically applicable.

5. Renin Activity:

- Normal Range: The normal range for renin activity varies depending on the laboratory and the patient's sodium intake.
- Interpretation:

- High renin activity in the presence of low aldosterone levels can suggest primary adrenal insufficiency.
- Critical Values:
  - Not typically applicable.

6. Electrolytes:

- Normal Range:
  - Sodium: 135-145 mmol/L
  - Potassium: 3.5-5.0 mmol/L
  - Chloride: 98-106 mmol/L
- Interpretation:
  - Hyponatremia (low sodium) and hyperkalemia (high potassium) can occur in adrenal insufficiency due to impaired aldosterone production.
- Critical Values:
  - Severe electrolyte imbalances can be life-threatening and require immediate medical attention.

Important Considerations:

- Reference Ranges: Reference ranges can vary slightly between laboratories. It's essential to interpret test results in conjunction with clinical findings and other laboratory tests.
- Interfering Factors: Certain medications, medical conditions, and laboratory techniques can affect test results.
- Healthcare Provider Interpretation: Always consult with your healthcare provider to interpret test results and discuss appropriate treatment options.

Emergency Protocol

An adrenal crisis is characterized by severe symptoms such as low blood pressure, shock, and altered mental status. Here's a comprehensive checklist to guide you through an adrenal crisis:

1. Recognize the Signs and Symptoms:

- Severe fatigue
- Nausea and vomiting

- Abdominal pain
- Dehydration
- Low blood pressure
- Rapid heart rate
- Confusion
- Loss of consciousness

2. Immediate Action:

- Call Emergency Services (911 or local emergency number): Immediately seek emergency medical attention.
- Administer Emergency Hydrocortisone: If you have a prescribed emergency injection of hydrocortisone, administer it as directed by your healthcare provider.
- Monitor Vital Signs: Check blood pressure, heart rate, and respiratory rate.
- Position the Person: Place the person in a comfortable position, preferably lying down with their legs elevated.
- Reassure the Person: Stay calm and reassure the person until emergency medical help arrives.

3. Hospital Treatment:

- Intravenous Fluids: To restore blood volume and correct electrolyte imbalances.
- High-Dose Hydrocortisone: To rapidly increase cortisol levels.
- Monitoring: Close monitoring of vital signs, blood glucose levels, and electrolyte levels.
- Additional Medications: As needed to treat specific symptoms or complications.

4. Post-Crisis Care:

- Gradual Tapering of Steroids: Under the supervision of a healthcare provider, slowly reduce the dosage of hydrocortisone to avoid rebound adrenal insufficiency.
- Follow-up Care: Schedule regular check-ups with your endocrinologist to monitor your condition and adjust medication as needed.
- Stress Management: Implement stress-reducing techniques to minimize the risk of future crises.
- Medical Alert Bracelet: Wear a medical alert bracelet or necklace to inform healthcare

providers of your condition in case of an emergency.

Additional Tips:

- Know Your Triggers: Be aware of factors that can trigger an adrenal crisis, such as illness, injury, or significant stress.
- Carry Emergency Medication: Always carry your emergency hydrocortisone injection with you.
- Educate Loved Ones: Teach family and friends about adrenal insufficiency and how to recognize and respond to an adrenal crisis.
- Regularly Review Your Emergency Plan: Update your emergency plan as needed to ensure it remains effective.

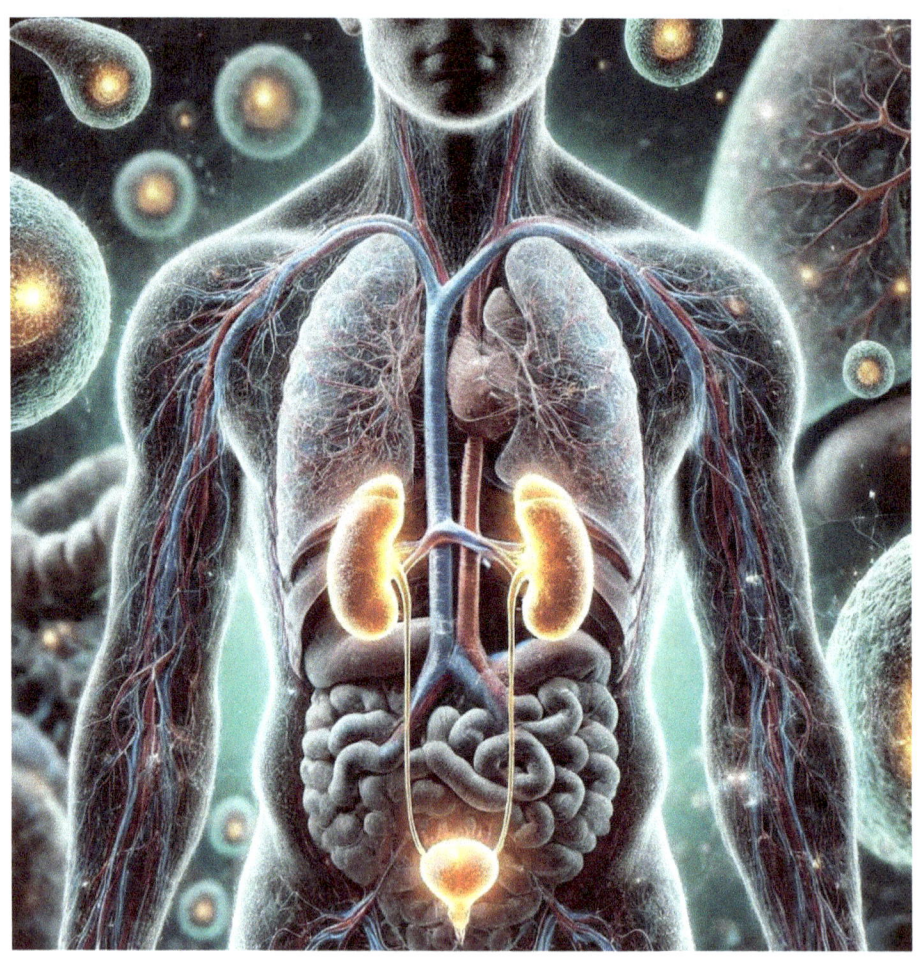

www.ingramcontent.com/pod-product-compliance
Lightning Source LLC
Chambersburg PA
CBHW062322220526
45469CB00008B/2595